Weight Loss
for
Wimps

Lose Your Belly Fat, Look Younger
And
Get Healthy, Sexy and Thin

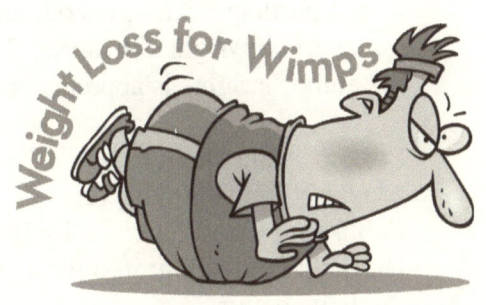

Kevin C. Myers

BlueChip Press, LLC

Published by BlueChip Press, LLC
5729 Lebanon Rd. Suite 144-204
Frisco, Texas 75034, USA

http://www.weightloss4wimps.com

Editor: Anita Davies:
adaviesediting@gmail.com
Publishing Consultant: Emily Hill, A.V.
Harrison Publishing: info@AVHarrison-Publishing.com
Cover Design: Tatiana Villa:
villatat@gmail.com

Cartoon Character: Ron Leishman:
ron@toonaday.com

Disclaimer: Weight Loss for Wimps™
The publisher, BlueChip Press LLC and the
author Kevin C. Myers are not medical
professionals and therefore we strongly
encourage you to see your physician before
starting any exercise or nutrition program. If
you have been sedentary, are overweight or
have high cholesterol, high blood pressure or
diabetes, you should have a complete physical
examination.

The advice and suggestions contained herein are
for educational purposes and are not intended to
be a substitute for advice provided by your
health care provider.

All forms of exercise pose some inherent risk;
readers are advised to take full responsibility for
their safety and to know their physical
limitations. Always ask for instruction and
assistance when using weight lifting equipment.

Dedication

To my lovely wife and lifelong sweetheart Sharon, your support on this project has been so important to me; thank you for your patience (and great cooking too)! To my daughter Nicole and her husband Aaron, I am so proud of both of you for all that you do and for your many accomplishments. And to my youngest daughter Tiffany… you are an incredible kid and I am so proud of you for using your amazing talents to help the poor people in Mozambique – come home soon!

Acknowledgements

Thanks so much to my publishing consultant Emily Hill and editor Anita Davies; you guys found and killed all of the many manuscript Gremlins and have otherwise provided invaluable support. And a special thanks to my friends who took the time to actually read the book and provide great editorial comments – Nicole Emerson, Tim Pinson, Lisa Bealhen, Sherry Ward, Ginette Laurin, Tim Lee and Michelle Poteet.

WHAT READERS ARE SAYING ABOUT *WEIGHT LOSS FOR WIMPS*

"Kevin is a magician! He transforms your thinking by weaving in success tools, skills, and motivation with specific <u>action steps</u> that will literally drop the weight for you. This book is AWESOME and I highly recommend it to ensure your success."
Lori L. Shemek, Ph.D., CNC, CLC; Health Expert for the #1 ABC Show "*Good Morning Texas*;" Creator of the *Nutrinetics*™ program and the *Health Attraction System*™

"I thought this was going to be another ho-hum, eat your vegetables diet book...boy was I wrong. This book is fabulous! For the first time I learned to identify my own bad habits and best of all, how to stop them myself. Great story telling. You kept me engaged and entertained at the same time. I haven't enjoyed a health book this much since reading Dr. Oz's **You on a Diet.*"***
Michelle P. – Austin, TX

"I really think that Kevin has a refreshing perspective on weight loss. I love the personal stories and could really relate to his struggles. The action steps in this book were extremely

helpful in preparing for my lifestyle change. I used the South Beach diet plan in conjunction with this book and have lost 30 pounds in 3 months!"
Emma B. – Juneau, AK

"As a personal trainer, this book will be a fantastic resource not only for me, but especially for my clients. This is the 'unfair advantage' I've been looking for! Great job Kevin!"
Kay Chumbley – Personal Trainer, Frisco, TX

Contents

Preface   **14**

Introduction – Setting the Table   **28**
- Obesity Gone Wild
- The Perfect Storm
- Hoodwinkia and Other "Miracle Pills"
- You Don't Need Another Hollywood Diet Book

Part 1: Preparing Your Mind for Incredible Weight Loss Success

Chapter One   **46**
Paying the Price of Admission
- Losing Weight Is Forrest Gump Simple, Right?
- The Mystery of Diet Success or Failure - Solved
- Bad Habits - The Most Powerful Force in the Universe
- What's It Going to Take?
- Success Step One

Chapter Two   **57**
Have You Reached Your Tipping Point?

- Your New Year's Resolution – How Did That Work Out?
- The Tipping Point Moment
- Capture the Power of Your Emotions
- Ready, Fire, Aim – You're Not Ready Yet
- Success Step Two

Chapter Three   **68**
Lifestyle Breakout™ – The Cornerstone Strategy

- Overview of the Lifestyle Breakout Strategy
- The Status Quo (Wimpdom) Is Not Your Friend
- Discover the Real Reason You Want to Be Thin
- Imagine You…Strutting Your Stuff
- Believe in the Big Dream
- Success Step Three

Chapter Four   **83**
Making YOU Priority #1

- After the Dog, Honey, Of Course You're #1
- Give Yourself Permission To Be #1

- The Healthy Obsession – All Day, Every Day
- Success Step Four

Chapter Five   **91**
Setting Your Weight Loss Goal
- When Twenty Lbs Isn't Good Enough
- What's Your Perfect Weight?
- All In – Go For the Gold and an Extraordinary Life
- Break It Down – One Month At a Time
- Success Step Five

Part 2: Tools and Tactics for Winning Every Battle

Chapter Six   **100**
You've Got Powerful Obstacles – Knowing Your Enemies
- Chalk Talk – The Big Picture
- The Big Four Bad Boys
- Can You Win Every Battle?
- How To Cheat Successfully – *No Fear*™ Technique
- Success Step Six

Chapter Seven   **110**
Tactics for Dealing with Excuses
- Excuses Are a Dime a Dozen

- Dead On Arrival Excuses
- No Where to Run, No Where to Hide
- Success Step Seven

Chapter Eight   **125**
Tactics for Dealing with Emotional Eating
- Emotional Eating Basics
- Uncomfortable Emotions and Uncomfortable Triggers
- The *I Learn*™ To End Emotional Eating Technique
- Identify Your Emotional Eating Behaviors
- Listen to Your Emotional Signals and Triggers
- Experience the Emotion – Go to Your Inner Sanctuary
- Analyze Your Options and Take Action
- Relief Valve
- Nurture a New Relationship With Food
- *I Love Good Food* ™Philosophy
- Success Step Eight

Chapter Nine   **150**
Tactics for Dealing with Stress
- Stress 101
- The Stress-Eating Connection
- Stress Coping Skills

- Deflate Your Self-Inflicted Lifestyle Stress
- Success Step Nine

Chapter Ten   **162**
Tactics for Dealing with Hunger
- The Special Powers of Hunger
- Diet Industry Malpractice
- How I Discovered Hunger Is My Friend
- Tactics for Dealing With Real Hunger – *Hunger Is Good Philosophy*™
- Fighting Real Hunger With Real Food
- Tactics For Dealing With Fake Hunger
- Circling the Wagons
- Success Step Ten

Part 3: Food – Eat, Eat, Eat!

Chapter Eleven   **176**
The Best Weight Loss Diet in the World
- Commercial Diet Programs
- The Evils of Our Western Diet
- In Search of the Perfect Diet
- 10 Abraham Lincoln Eating Rules™
- How Many Calories Should I Eat?
- Success Step Eleven

Chapter Twelve   **196**
The Simple Lifestyle Changes That Saved My Life
- Life Is Not a Bowl of Cherries
- Simple Healthy Meals…For Dummies Like Me!
- Portion Control Made Easy
- Exercise – Completing the Trifecta
- Success Step Twelve

Part 4: Rocket Fuel

Chapter Thirteen   **208**
Exercise – Get That Butt Moving!
- I Hate to Exercise
- Oh No…You've Got "Man-Boobs?!"
- Can You Spare Fifteen Minutes For a Workout?
- The *Wimps Intensive*™ Protocol
- *Wimps Weight Lifting*
- Working Out at Home
- Success Step Thirteen

Chapter Fourteen   **229**
For Those Who Will Settle for Nothing Less Than Outrageous Success
- Public Accountability
- The Hot, Sexy Personal Trainer

- Weight Loss Coaching
- What's the Score – Monitoring Your Progress
- Success Step Fourteen

Appendix: Master Plan   **241**
- Weight Loss for Wimps™ Tools
- Weight Loss for Wimps™ Success Steps

About the Author   **258**

Preface

Welcome Wimps!

I LOVE WIMPS because I have been one too, for most of my life. Take a good look at yourself and see if you have any of these characteristics: a long list of excuses, blaming others, no motivation, no mental toughness, yo-yo dieting, occasional to constant whining, frequently go to all-you-can-eat buffets, always start the New Year with a diet resolution.

The good news is, this behavior and mental outlook is about to change for you, permanently. You will soon become a "former Wimp."

I'm Pumped Up and Excited for <u>You</u>!

I am very happy today, because right now, I have the chance to dramatically impact a life … <u>your life,</u> and lead you to the no wimp lifestyle.

Yep, I have a <u>big vision</u> and a <u>big promise</u>.

My big vision is to contribute to helping solve the worldwide pandemic of obesity or Globesity, by helping <u>you</u> and my other readers around the world - *one mind and one heart at a time*.

The focus of this book is passing on to <u>you</u> the *attitudes, implementation skills and action plan* that are necessary to solve, once and for all, *your* weight problems. And my <u>big promise</u> is simply this:

Open your mind and open your heart
Obtain the knowledge and learn the skills
Implement what you learn, that is the key
You <u>will</u> reach the weight you want to be

Regardless of your age, wealth, social status, or sex, your current weight is a significant issue in your life. Otherwise, you wouldn't have purchased this book.

Give yourself *permission* to focus on this problem and if you do, I can help you solve it, permanently.

Are you a little skeptical?

You should be, so let's have a little conversation...

In Search of the Secret
You've been on "umpteen" diets before this, right? Of course. We've all been on dozens of diets and they just don't seem to work out for us, especially in the long run. We may lose some weight here and there, particularly if we can get past the first week of hell.

But then, *"it"* happens and we quickly go back to our regular habits, gain the weight back and maybe more. The cycle is never ending.

What is *"it"?*

"It" is life.

The daily grind of kids, spouse, school, pressures at your crappy job, your pathetic boss, your long commute. Or maybe you recently lost your job in this horrific worldwide recession. You know, the stuff we *all* have to put up with each and every day.

In the last few days or weeks, something else has happened in your life to "trigger" you to once again seek help in getting your weight under control and begin living a healthy lifestyle.

The problem is; you have no real confidence that you're <u>really</u> going to accomplish anything. Deep down, you're skeptical and probably thinking that in the end it's probably going to be, "Same story, different verse."

Stay with me now, because things are going to change, <u>big time</u>!

I'm about to reveal to you, exactly what you've been looking for - the secret sauce, the magic bullet, the holy grail that has alluded you thus far - exactly how to lose all the weight you need to lose, permanently.

In fact, I'm going to share this "closely guarded secret" with you right now, upfront. So, theoretically, you won't even have to read the rest of the book.

Here it comes…

"Cut the Crap and Burn the Fat!"

Yep, that's it.

Eliminate the junk food, eat more fruits and vegetables and move around a bit more than you do now, and you will lose weight. Lots and lots of weight.

A simple Albert Einstein's thermodynamic equation: *Burn more calories than you take in and you will lose all the weight you want.*

But, of course, you already knew that.

Now, for the rest of the story…

Connecting the Dots

I've had a weight problem for almost my entire life. There have been only three relatively brief periods when I have been at my ideal weight:

1. When I was born
2. When I completed military basic training (officer candidate school)
3. Now, after losing 88 lbs and keeping it off for almost four years

The first two instances don't count because I didn't really have any input. It just happened "naturally."

A couple of years ago, at 6' 2", I weighed 285 lbs, was diagnosed with Type 2 diabetes, was popping five nitroglycerin pills a day to relieve my chest pain, plus blood pressure pills, etc. I wore extra-extra large (2XX) shirts and had a 44" waist. In short, I was out of control and knew I was going to assume room temperature at any moment. I thought about that every day.

My wife and I were living the good life in Costa Rica. We'd spent about three and a half years down there, living in a small beach community.

One day, I was in San Jose (capital city) and decided to fly back to the beach town where we lived. This was a short forty minute flight on a small eighteen seat commuter plane that would save me from four hours of pounding in a car. All I had with me was a shoulder bag, which held a laptop and some clothes.

I went to the airport and started the check-in process:

"Please step on the scales with your carry-on bag...
I'm sorry sir, but you will need to
purchase a second ticket.
Your weight is well in excess of our criteria."

Needless to say, I was *furious*. My Spanish cussing vocabulary was fairly limited, but I got my message across.

In the end, I paid for the extra seat and vowed to <u>never</u> fly that airline again. The embarrassment and humiliation was excruciating. Those bas#%!@! were never going to get another dime out of me!

But then, on the short flight home I got to thinking… "You idiot… don't you think it's time to lose the extra weight you're hauling around?"

Now, I was pissed off at myself and vowed to do something about it. I was at a *"tipping point."*

Of course, I went on a "diet." I started cutting back on this and that, small portions of everything. It was hell and I was miserable, but I began losing weight. In fact, I lost about 20 lbs over the next couple of months.

But then, "it" happened and I started cheating more often, making excuses to myself and losing confidence that I could actually do this. The weight loss stalled completely, and I started gaining back a few pounds. Here we go again - another failed attempt.

In retrospect, I didn't appreciate the strength of the bad habits I had accumulated over a lifetime or how difficult it was going to be to break these habits. And I certainly didn't give any thought to this issue before I started the "diet."

Then, one of my daughters came to visit and observed my weakened condition. One day, in a private moment only fathers and daughters can share, she said,

*"Dad, I love you very much and
I don't want you to die on me.*

*Please get yourself healthy again.
I need you to walk me
down the aisle someday."*

That night, after everyone was asleep, I began reflecting on my life, my health situation and my daughter's heartfelt plea. The tears came and I started fantasizing about what it would *feel* like to be thin again - going to my daughter's wedding, walking her down the aisle, tall, thin and proud. This was my *"**white hot moment.**"* A highly emotional moment when I *finally* realized I had to take massive and irreversible action to correct my situation... I knew that I *had* to do it and that I *could* do it, and that I was *going* to do it, no matter what.

I began to understand that just "going on a diet" was not going to work. I needed a *system* that would help me work through not just "what to eat" and "how much to eat."

I knew instinctively that I had to fight this battle *in my mind*. And I knew that *I* had to fight this battle alone - or so I thought.

Men don't ask directions when they get lost driving. And they sure as hell don't buy diet books or go to weekly group meetings (unless they are very, very smart!). We know what needs to be done (eat less, exercise more) so it's just a matter of doing it.

Well, as usual, it didn't work out so well.

Sure, I had lost the 20 lbs but kept slipping, stalling and cheating almost daily. Twenty lbs was good, but not good enough when you need to lose 100 lbs.

Feeling sorry for myself one day, I said to my wife in passing, "… maybe I should go to a fat camp somewhere." Of course, I had absolutely no intention of *ever* going to one. I knew nothing about them and didn't want to know. After all, I *knew* what had to be done.

My wife, bless her heart, had other ideas. Within two days, in passing, she informed me "… you're booked on a flight to Hilton Head, SC on Saturday… you'll be gone for three weeks."

"What? There is no way I'm going to some lame fat camp. Period. That was just a joke the other day."

"Well it's not a joke now, buddy…you're going, so start packing."

Deep down, I knew I needed some help. I just wouldn't man-up and admit it.

Long story short, I went. I lost another 17 lbs. Woo-Hoo! But, at $10,000 total cost for the three weeks, that works out to be about $588 per pound lost - ouch!

Going to a weight loss camp is just like what you see on the TV show ***Biggest Loser***. It's an artificial environment where you are fed and exercised by others.

When you get home, you're on your own, and if you're not careful, back to square one.

As a side note, about 35% of the people at the camp were "repeat offenders" i.e. had been to camp multiple times. In fact, my roommate was on his eighth visit and still at 300 lbs. With a little help and encouragement from me, he lost 22 lbs at camp and went home and lost another 60 for a total of 80 lbs and reached his ideal weight. Unfortunately, he later gained it all back.

Would I recommend that you go to a weight loss camp?

If you can afford the time and the expense, absolutely. But it is not a panacea and _will not_, by itself solve your weight problem.

The biggest benefit of going to camp was that I _gave myself_ permission to make regaining my health and losing weight the _number one priority in my life_.

When I returned home to Costa Rica, I felt great but still had about 50 lbs to lose in order to reach my goal weight of 197 lbs. I couldn't stop now - I had to go all the way.

Now what?

I had all of the "how to" information I would ever need:

I knew what to eat…
I knew how much to eat…
I knew what not to eat…
I knew the importance of exercise and weight training…

But now that I was back in "real life", I was immediately faced with major obstacles for which I was _not_ prepared and had _no_ solutions for:

- Creating excuses for being fat and not staying on a sensible eating plan
- Wanting to use food to make me feel better when I was emotionally upset but not actually hungry
- Wanting to eat in reaction to the pressures of work or the stress of daily living
- Dealing with real physical hunger for the first time ever
- Making the time available in my daily schedule and staying motivated to exercise on a daily basis

This is where the rubber meets the road - the daily battles that go on *in the mind* that must be fought and won every day, day in and day out.

I had to develop a plan, a strategy and tactics for fighting *each* of these mental wars. I did and the end result of this effort is found in the remaining pages of this book.

It turns out that 90% of your weight loss success will come from acquiring the proper mindset and having a plan in place to fight and win these mental battles. And you must think through these issues **BEFORE** you start your eating plan.

Over time and through trial and error, I was able to accomplish everything I wanted. I reached my ideal weight, shrunk my waist to 34" and now wear a size large shirt.

I can't begin to describe how it *feels* to be healthy, sexy and thin. It is incredible beyond belief and something I want *you* to feel. It will change your life in ways that you may not even realize at this point. Follow me and I will teach you the system.

But before we get started, you need to do some serious self-talk.

- Know and *believe* that this is something *you can achieve*, regardless of your current weight or past experience with diets.

- Know and *believe* that you *deserve* to be successful in losing the weight and obtaining all the incredible benefits that will come your way as a result.

- Dream big and let your emotions bubble to the surface. Visualize detailed and specific scenarios about how you will look and feel at your ideal weight.

- Make a commitment to yourself to go "all in." This is the last time you will ever need to go through this process. You will never be a wimp again. Period.

In the words of the great American hero Todd Beamer on United Airlines Flight 93:

"Are you guys ready? Let's roll!"

INTRODUCTION

Setting The Table

OBESITY GONE WILD
Did you know that right now, today, we are in the middle of a health crisis of historic and epidemic proportions?

No, it's not Swine Flu or heart disease…

It's obesity.

Depending on your age, look around at your friends and family or strangers at the mall or at school… and people may look pretty normal.

Other people look around and notice that just about everyone is overweight…ok, fat.

In just the last 30 to 40 years, obesity worldwide has *exploded*.
In 2008, according to the Center for Disease Control (CDC), about 65% of the adults in America are either overweight or obese (BMI index of > 25 i.e. at least 25% over their ideal weight). *That is two out of every three people.*

In 1960, the CDC numbers show that only 33% of the adults in America were overweight or obese. That's a whopping 100% increase, but it gets worse.
If you look at just obesity (BMI index of >30), the numbers are even more staggering. In 1960

the percentage of the adult population in America who were obese was less than 10% (9.7%). In 2008, the percentage was about 32% - a *230% increase. Wow!*

And it's not just us "fat cat" Americans, Canadians, Europeans or other so-called Western countries. The World Health Organization (WHO) estimates that 60% of men and 50% of women are now overweight or obese in such diverse countries as China, Argentina, Turkey, Mexico and Russia. In 2000, the United Nations reported that for the first time ever the number of people suffering from over-nutrition (overweight) had officially surpassed those suffering from malnutrition.

What about our children? I can't begin to describe the fear, hurt and pain I feel for our children. Setting aside the grotesque social insults, isolation, and emotional trauma our fat kids experience and endure at school and as young adults, their health is also in crisis:

A recent study in the New England Journal of Medicine (2005) reported that our children and teens are so fat that their life expectancy has been cut by up to 5 years; the first reduction since the early 1800's.

The implications of this are outrageous:

Our kids will be the first generation ever who are <u>not</u> expected to live as long as their parents.

This is pathetic.

Something big is going on… something *insidious*… a game changer that has affected the world… and something nobody seems to have a handle on…

What the heck has happened?!

You need to know the answer to this question, because until you *really* understand what has happened to <u>*you*</u> and everyone else, you will have a difficult time fixing the problem in <u>*your*</u> life.

The Perfect Storm
The answer to this question is complex and has taken me over a year to figure out. I'm not going to bore you with all the details (although they are fascinating) because my job is to teach by simplification.

It boils down to the simultaneous timing of two primary factors (and several secondary factors) that have led to the "perfect storm". The result has been the destruction of our collective health:

1. Significant decrease in our daily physical activity

2. Explosive growth (worldwide) in consumption of processed foods in our Western Diet resulting in a dramatic increase in our daily consumption of cheap, nutritionally empty, high density calories, *particularly high fructose corn syrup (HFCS).*

The first factor is obvious and really needs no further explanation. We all know that physical education has all but disappeared from our schools, as adults we fight to get the parking spot closest to the entry door, we watch way too much television, and we never exercise on purpose. In short, we are a collective society of wimpy couch potatoes and inactive slugs. And we all know what needs to be done to fix this problem (discussed further in Chapter 13).

The second factor may seem obvious in that we intuitively know we are eating too many calories. But what is not obvious or widely known by the public is the *sudden appearance in 1980* of an insidious new substance, never before known to man – **_high fructose corn syrup_** – that is now a dominant component of the Western diet food supply.

I discovered this little bit of critical information buried on page 102 of a book hardly anyone has ever heard of: *The Omnivore's Dilemma*. This book written by Michael Pollan, a University of California Berkeley professor and is perhaps the most important book of our time written on the history of agriculture and food supply. His follow up book, *In Defense of Food*, is equally important and highly recommended.

Fructose is of course, a natural sugar found in many fruits and some vegetables in relatively low concentrations. But the clever, nerdy food scientists discovered a way to refine a highly concentrated form of this sweet tasting carbohydrate from a government subsidized cheap source – corn.

Introduced to the market in 1980, each of us now consumes the calorie packed substance to the tune of *66 lbs per year*. Much of this is consumed in soft drinks because Coca-Cola and other brands started using this source of sugar because it was cheaper than sugarcane. By 1984 they switched entirely to corn syrup. But note that this has not replaced our sugar usage…

since 1985 our per capita sugar consumption has increased from 128 lbs to 168 lbs per person (31% increase).

We went from zero to about 13.2 teaspoons per day per person of HFCS. The average American drinks the equivalent of a 12 pack of Cola each week. Each 12 ounce can of Coke contains 140 calories and 39 grams of sugar (all of it HFCS).

However, it goes way, way beyond soft drinks. The food geeks have incorporated this little monster in just about every form of processed food you can think of - chips, crackers, ketchup, mayonnaise, ice cream, pizza sauce, peanut butter, ham, deli meats, spaghetti sauce, yogurt, hot dogs, salad dressing, sausage, coffee creamers, bread, and the 17,000 *new* fake foods they create and put on the grocery shelves *every year*. Read the labels, you'll see it everywhere. For a list of common commercial food brands containing HFCS, please visit this site: http://tinyurl.com/HFCS-list

Isn't it interesting that the introduction of HFCS coincides *almost exactly* with CDC statistics that show Americans increased their daily calorie intake by about 15% during the period of 1971 to 2000. On average that's around an *extra 250 calories per day.*

Going deeper into the CDC numbers, it gets worse…**particularly for <u>women</u>**. The study found women increased their daily calorie consumption 22% or an *extra 335 calories per day*. Why? The study concludes it is "mainly due to an increase in carbohydrate consumption." In my opinion: HFCS

And guess where all these extra calories go?

If you're a man, they turn into fat and are stored around your belly (primarily).

If you're a woman, they turn into fat and are stored around your butt (golo if you're Greek!) and legs (primarily).

An increase of 250 calories per day results in about 25 lbs per year. And 335 extra calories per day results in about 33.5 extra lbs per year.

Many point to the explosive growth of fast food restaurants and the invention of the super-sized meal. Certainly these factors have added significantly to the problem. Because many of these fast food items contain loads of HFCS; and super-sizing means you're eating a lot more of them at each meal. Check out this site for fast

foods containing HFCS:
http://tinyurl.com/HFCS-fastfood

HFCS is loved by food manufactures because it is cheap, adds addictive taste to many food items, provides filler, stabilizes foods and increases shelf life. And best of all, consumers like you and I have no idea it even exist!

High fructose corn syrup - an innocent sounding little sugar refined from corn, that has changed the world.

Hoodwinkia and Other "Miracle Pills"
Wouldn't it be great if you could just take a magic pill and all your excess weight disappeared almost overnight?

Fantasies are the fuel of life because some of them (the realistic ones) can actually come true. But forget about the magic pill - it's just not going to happen.

I have a certain philosophy about appetite suppressants like *Hoodia* and fat absorption pills like *Alli*. Regardless of whether or not they actually "work," in my view they are preventing you from transforming your mind and body to a healthy place.

Let me ask you a couple of simple but serious questions that I want you to really think about... is that ok?

- *Is it possible that you sometimes, or maybe oftentimes, eat when you are not really hungry?*

For most of us the answer is absolutely _yes_. That being the case, what benefit is there to a pill that suppresses your appetite but then you eat when you're not hungry anyway? You are only fooling yourself.

- *Would you pay $50 for a one month supply of Alli or any other fat absorption pill when your weight loss benefit is only 3 lbs per year compared to a sensible diet and exercise program?*

One of the most prestigious hospitals/clinics in the U.S. is the world famous Mayo Clinic. The 3lbs per year benefit is the conclusion made by Dr. Donald Hensrud, M.D., a preventative medicine and nutrition specialist at the Mayo Clinic in Minnesota. You can read his report about Alli here:
http://tinyurl.com/Alli-MayoClinic

I'm a strong advocate for rebuilding and strengthening your body through diet, exercise and with certain vitamins, minerals and natural health supplements. I frequently recommend supplements to my clients, depending on their unique needs.

The point is, you are going to have to do this "weight loss thing" yourself, not with magic pills. It's all about *Attitude, Skills and Action*.

You Don't Need Another Hollywood Diet Book

The last thing the world needs is another high profile diet book. With 25,000 diet books currently in publication, don't you suppose *somebody* has it right?

The truth is, many of the diet books out there are fantastic - brilliant even. There are many very smart people who have created excellent diet books with great tasting recipes, shopping lists and styles of eating... South Beach Diet, Atkins Diet, Zone Diet and several excellent pre-made meal programs like Jenny Craig®, and NutriSystems® (among others).

And guess what - they *all work* because at the basic level, they all reduce your *overall caloric intake* to a level that is below your caloric burn rate.

A recent study published in the New England Journal of Medicine compared the weight loss results of over 800 people using three styles of diets: one a low-fat, one a low carb, and the other a high protein diet. Each was designed to cut 750 calories a day and included 90 minutes of exercise per week (not much!). The result – all three groups lost *exactly the same amount of weight* (average of 13lbs over six months). Their earth-shattering conclusion:

"It's simply a matter of calories."

So, why is it that we voraciously consume new diet books each year, as if the "final solution" has just been invented?

It's because so many of us have failed in our previous attempts at losing weight and we are *hoping* that this "new diet" will work for us. I understand this first hand because we've all been there and *without hope there is only unhappiness and despair*. At least those of us who are buying the books are making an attempt to do something about our situation…just like *you are* with this book.

Selecting a specific diet (eating) program is a very personal and very individualized decision. One size does not fit all. One must consider food preferences, culture, and health issues among other factors.

If you haven't guessed already, I prefer a real food, whole food (organic), lower carbohydrate style of eating. I include some fruit, lots of different vegetables and a protein i.e. seafood, freshwater fish, chicken or some grass fed beef. But that's just me.

The overriding concept is to significantly lower caloric intake so that your body can start consuming all the excess fat you have accumulated. It's that simple.

Overview of the Weight Loss for Wimps™ System

My approach to helping you is something different.

Based on my own experiences and observing many others, I've discovered that what people *really* want is a comprehensive systems approach to the problem of losing weight that focuses on the weak link – *the mental aspects of weight loss*. This is the area where most people mess it up, usually during the first week…two weeks if you're Superman!

The key components of the *Weight Loss for Wimps* ™ *System* can be summarized as follows:

Part I: Preparing Your Mind for Incredible Weight Loss Success

- Understanding that losing weight is simple, but not easy. Bad eating behavior and habits are difficult to break. You have to be willing to pay the price. Covered in Chapter One.

- Understanding that to be successful in losing weight, you have to experience an emotional *"tipping point"* – a trigger event that you *feel* in your heart (pain) that provides a stimulus to get you to at least start *thinking* about taking action. Covered in Chapter Two.

- Understanding that you <u>*must*</u> dig deep into your heart and emotions to uncover the most important reason(s) for <u>*why*</u> you want to lose weight (motivation); and then create a detailed and specific vision, the <u>big dream</u>, of what you will *look* like and how you will *feel* at your ideal weight (benefits). Imagine <u>you</u> - <u>strutting your stuff</u>! Covered in Chapter Three.

- Understanding that no matter how busy you are with life, you cannot succeed at weight loss UNTIL you make the decision that your health and happiness are moved to the front of the line – Making <u>you priority number one</u>. Covered in Chapter Four.

- Understanding that to achieve your perfect weight goal and obtain the maximum benefits of being thin, you MUST go "all in". Go For the Gold and an <u>extraordinary life</u>. Covered in Chapter Five.

Part II: Tools and Tactics for Winning Every Battle

- Introduction to your enemies – excuses, emotional eating, stress and physical hunger and the concept that you *must* prepare a battle plan *in advance* of starting your new eating plan. Covered in Chapter Six.

- Specific tactics (skills) that you can use to win the battles with each of the mental enemies you will face each day. Covered in Chapters Seven to Ten.

Part III: Food – Eat, Eat, Eat!

- The best weight loss diet in the world is identified with critical criteria necessary for long-term success. Covered in Chapter 11.

- A description of the eating program I follow which has allowed me to lose 88 lbs and keep it off for almost four years. No calorie counting required! Chapter 12.

Part IV: Rocket Fuel

- Accelerate your weight loss progress and your health with a consistent exercise program. You don't need weights or a health club membership but you may want to consider one anyway. Chapter 13.

- Accelerate your weight loss progress with public accountability. This could come from family, friends, co-workers, a coach or personal trainer. But you need to be very careful with your selections. Hang with the wrong people and you're doomed. Chapter 14.

- Accelerate your weight loss progress by keeping score – monitor your progress on a regular basis so that you can make adjustments to your eating and exercise programs. Chapter 14.

IMPORTANT NOTE:

I have designed the *Weight Loss for Wimps™ System* to be fully implemented after completing the 14 Success Steps discussed in the 14 Chapters. Furthermore, I have created a *Weight Loss for Wimps™ Quick Start Guide, Daily Journal and Implementation Protocol* wherein the 14 Success Steps are carefully completed *over a seven day period*. This allows you to get the *mindset mojo skills* and techniques needed to achieve outrageous success with your health and weight loss goals.

For a *free* copy of the **Quick Start Guide, Daily Journal and Implementation Protocol** simply go to http://www.wimpdailyjournal.com and you'll be able to download a copy.

PART ONE

**PREPARING YOUR MIND
FOR INCREDIBLE
WEIGHT LOSS
SUCCESS**

CHAPTER ONE

PAYING THE PRICE OF ADMISSION

LOSING WEIGHT IS Forrest Gump Simple, Right?
We've already covered the Forrest Gump Simple, works every time, and can't miss, absolutely guaranteed, proven beyond all doubt, certified solutions to losing weight:

- "Cut the crap and burn the fat"
- "Burn more calories than you take in"
- "It's simply a matter of calories"

It doesn't matter what diet program or style of eating you ultimately choose, it all boils down to calories in and calories out - simple.

If losing weight is so simple, why are we all so fat?
If losing weight is so simple, we'd all be thin!

Losing weight *is* simple - but not *easy*.

And that is the catch. Not only is it *not easy*, it's downright difficult. No fluff here. I put it right up there with quitting smoking, which for me was equally as difficult as losing weight. You've got to really, really *want* to do it. And you've got to prepare yourself mentally for the challenge.

The message I want you to understand is this...

There is a price to pay for weight loss success

There will be moments where you will feel very uncomfortable...

There will be moments where you will feel very hungry...

There will be moments where you will feel strong cravings...

There will be moments where you will feel emotionally upset...

There will be moments where you will feel totally stressed out...

There will be moments where you will feel like giving up...

There will be moments where you will feel deprived...

There will be moments where you will feel it's not worth the pain...
There will be moments where you will feel angry at your loved ones...

There will be moments where you will feel angry at the world...

During my weight loss journey, I experienced all of these physical and emotional sensations, thoughts and more, *particularly in the early weeks*. It can be like being on a wild roller coaster ride.

You too will experience these negative thoughts, feelings, and emotions at times. The feelings can be fleeting or intense but mostly they are brief... just understand that its part of the price you must be willing to pay to achieve weight loss success.

My purpose here is to help you understand what the experience will be like, and to know that it's normal and to be expected.

Psychologists who have extensively studied people undertaking major changes in behavior such as eating habits or quitting smoking, have noted that those people, who have honestly contemplated the downsides before starting to implement the changes, were the most successful.

They understood and acknowledged the negatives, and decided they *wanted to do it anyway.*

The Mystery of Diet Success or Failure - Solved

It's no secret that about 90% of people who start a diet to lose weight will ultimately fail. In some cases, little to no weight is actually lost and in other cases a lot of weight is lost. Regardless, the weight is then regained very quickly.

Only 10% achieve their weight loss goal and maintain their desired weight permanently.

I know in my heart that right now, <u>at the moment you read this</u>, you are thinking… "I want to be in the 10% group… but… I don't know if I can really do it?"

Let me remove all doubt - work with me through this learning process and you <u>*will*</u> be a *<u>ten percenter!</u>*

So, the logical question at this point is…

"__Why__ do most people fail on a weight loss program?"

Failure leaves clues...

Hint: It is *not* lack of willpower...

I have extensively evaluated my own weight loss failures, talked with dozens of readers from around the world and studied reams of articles and books on the subject. There are many, many reasons suggested as the main reason for failure, all of which have some validity.

Nevertheless, I have crystallized my thinking on this and offer the following observation:

"The __number one__ cause of weight loss failure can almost __always__ be traced to the lack of a plan for dealing with the negative emotions experienced on a daily basis during the early weeks of the weight loss process."

__Key Concept__: Weight loss success or failure is about <u>emotions</u>. Dealing with negative emotions and focusing on positive ones. This is the process of *"getting your mindset mojo."*

Another misconception about "diets" is that they *don't work*. Several high profile weight loss programs and gurus make this claim, and then go on to sell their diet books or pre-packaged foods. These claims are clearly a marketing ploy, to entice serial dieters into their fold.

Of course diets work, if people learn how to focus their thoughts on the positive benefits they are achieving as they move towards their goal.

One big problem is one's *attitude* to the term "diet." For most people, the term has a negative meaning because a diet is something you must *endure* for a brief period of time. And after your endurance runs out (one week? three weeks?) you give up, wimp out and go back to your old eating habits.

"Whew! I'm sure glad that three weeks of hell is over!"

The successful weight loss *attitude* is…

"I'm not going on a diet. I'm permanently changing my eating habits and lifestyle. This is forever and I can't wait to become healthy, sexy and thin!"

Going on a diet is *very* stressful and that's the last thing you need to add to your busy life.

Changing your eating habits and lifestyle is an option you choose because it is exciting, invigorating and something you <u>want</u> to do, above all else.

Bad Habits – The Most Powerful Force in the Universe

The process of breaking your bad habits will trigger some or all of the "pain" discussed above …the price you <u>will</u> pay for weight loss success. So, what's the cause of all these negative feelings and emotions?

It's your efforts to break the bad habits you've accumulated over a lifetime. These include any action, inaction, thought pattern or behavior that you *know* is not moving you towards your goal of healthy weight loss.

Do you have any of these common bad habits?
- Eating generous amounts of calorie dense "comfort food"
- Frequently visiting fast-food and buffet style restaurants
- Never eating a real breakfast (coffee and donuts don't count)

- Eating on a fixed schedule even when you are not hungry
- Eating when you are upset, angry or stressed
- Cleaning your plate in seven minutes or less
- Eating your spouses or kids leftovers (personal favorite)
- Getting second or third helpings of your favorite dishes
- Drinking Cokes, beer, latte's or other sugar laden drinks on a daily basis
- Frequently eating large portions of white pasta, white rice or white bread
- Frequently buying snacks from vending machines or mini-markets
- Loading up on candy and buttered popcorn at the movies
- Eating ice cream, cookies, candy, cake or pie at least once a week
- Eating potato chips, corn chips, pretzels, or similar at least once a week
- Never or infrequently exercising on purpose
- Spending large chunks of your *free time* in front of the TV or computer

These are just a few bad habits. I'm sure you can add some others to your list?

Bad habits are the most powerful force in the universe, without question. And the process of breaking these habits and substituting healthy eating and lifestyle habits is the primary outcome we are seeking with the *Weight Loss for Wimps™ System.*

It's going to be challenging and it's going to be a source of a certain amount of emotional and even physical discomfort.

That's the _truth_.

What Is It Going To Take?

Success also leaves clues…

There are several key success principles and success implementation tactics that will be covered extensively in the following pages. All are extremely important components of the overall plan outlined in the *Weight Loss for Wimps™ System.*

The mindset of success will certainly include mental toughness, focus, determination, perseverance and desire coupled with a specific plan for handling the daily mental challenges.

But there is *one success clue* that I have found to be of **supreme importance**:

"The <u>number one</u> factor that will determine your weight loss success will be the level of emotional passion you develop around your <u>Big Dream</u>."

This passion for the vision of yourself, having already achieved your weight loss goal, will be the <u>unstoppable force</u> that will get you through the periods of pain that you will encounter.

This is part of developing your *mindset mojo* and will be discussed in great detail in Chapter Three.

But before you get there, you have to encounter something in your life that really *"rocks your world."* A significant emotional trigger or *tipping point* event that causes you to seriously consider breaking your bad habits. We'll get to that in Chapter Two.

Weight Loss for Wimps ™
Success Step One

Attitude: I know there is a price to pay to break my bad habits and I am willing to pay that price to reach my healthy weight loss goal

I am going to permanently change my eating habits and lifestyle because I want to, not because I should

Skills: I will get the Daily Journal at www.wimpdailyjournal.com and use this for my weight loss adventure

I will make a comprehensive list of all my bad habits – I know what they are!

Action: Pick two bad habits that you will focus on and eliminate *immediately*. Eliminate more as you learn the techniques to deal with negative emotions and learn to substitute healthy habits. Record these in your daily journal

CHAPTER TWO

HAVE YOU REACHED YOUR TIPPING POINT?

NEW YEAR'S RESOLUTION – How Did That Work Out?

Making one or more (typically three) New Year's resolutions is very common, worldwide. And the top three almost always includes weight loss, making more money and getting better organized.

Why not? Start fresh, do over, and turn the page…

How did your weight loss resolution work out for you this year? Or last year?

Recent studies estimate that about 55% of Americans make at least one resolution but after about three weeks, it's usually over. Roughly 90% of the people making resolutions fail to accomplish **any** of their goals. Does the 90-10 ratio sound familiar?

The problem is that most resolutions are made casually, with very little serious thought and certainly without any plan in mind. It's just a good idea at that particular moment…

"Sounds good honey, I'll help you lose weight. Cheers!"

There's no *emotional investment* or *commitment* in the process, just wishful thinking.

The Tipping Point
The term "tipping point" actually comes from the world of epidemiology but was popularized by Malcolm Gladwell in his best-selling book *The Tipping Point*. Gladwell applied the term to social phenomenon and describes how seemingly small changes or events can very suddenly gain momentum and then erupt and result in drastic societal change.

I like the term and have chosen to use it here to apply to an event that has happened or will happen to you, that causes a deep emotional reaction, which leads you to start thinking… *"I want to do something about my weight issue. I've had enough."*

Remember my tipping point, when I had to buy an extra seat on the airplane because I was too heavy? I think I had *blood shooting out of my eyes* at that moment! It got me very, very emotional. But most of all, it got me thinking about finally doing something to correct the problem I'd been avoiding all those years.

A tipping point can be like a bolt of lightning that really gets your emotions boiling. Or it can be a series of events over time that eventually will cause you to break down and decide you *want* do something about your situation. Usually it is something that makes you very angry, very hurt, very fearful or very sad.

In most cases, the stimulus is something you perceive externally and then internalize. Let's take a look at some examples from real life.

Relationships, Family and Friends

- Your husband slips up and tells the truth when you again ask the question…"Honey, do I look fat in these jeans?" (forgot his Pinocchio role)
- No one has asked for your phone number in three years
- You hear your friend trying to set you up on a blind date…*"He's smart, funny and has a great personality."*
- You overhear a neighborhood kid talking with your kid…*"Why is your Dad so fat?"*

- You get left alone at the nightclub again, after dutifully playing "wingman" for your friend
- Your spouse or partner hasn't shown any romantic interest in you for way too long...or maybe you realize it's *you* that has been in a state of "sexual radio silence" for a long time
- You're getting divorced, or will be shortly. The toxic relationship is coming to an end (sadly, but necessary) and you realize you will soon be alone
- You find yourself getting very jealous at social gatherings (or at work) when a well dressed, attractive woman walks in the room and you notice all the guys glancing in her direction. You're actually staring daggers at her. Then you find out she's actually older than you.

Health and Wellness

- You've been diagnosed with heart disease, diabetes and or other serious illness. You know your body will continue deteriorating unless you take immediate action
- A close friend, co-worker or family member just died suddenly from a heart attack

- You can't go skiing, play baseball or go bike riding with your kids or grandkids
- You can't go to the ballgames anymore because it's too difficult for you to hike across the parking lot and climb the stadium stairs
- You desperately want to start a family but your doctor has advised you that your weight may be too high to conceive. Or you've been diagnosed with the hormonal disorder PCOS (polycystic ovary syndrome; one in fifteen women have this condition and it can also be the *source* of your weight gain)

Work
- You've just been laid off at work in this lousy economy. You're fat, 42 and haven't had to interview for a new job in years
- You got passed over again for that dream job and know you've been working your butt off for it for years. You look around the company and realize most of the supervisors and managers are relatively thin. You suddenly suspect that weight bias may have played a role

- You're in the military, a policeman, a fireman or flight attendant…your boss just sent out another memo about weight management policies and expectations.

Upcoming Events
- You just got a posting on your Facebook page from your high school girlfriends that you haven't seen in 10 years; they expect you to be at the class reunion in July. You've only got five months
- You've got a wedding to go to - you're getting married, your son or daughter is getting married, or you've been asked to be part of the wedding ceremony, whatever - you're going - and you're worried sick about your appearance.

You get the idea. There are hundreds of combinations of these and many others. Can you relate to *any* of these scenarios? Are any of them occurring in your life right now? Are you *feeling* angry, upset, fearful or sad… how about jealous or envious? How about all of the above!

Good! Fantastic! Maybe you've reached **_your tipping point._**

<u>Key Point</u>: *Unless we are faced with a Major Emotional Event that brings about a sudden change in our wants, desires and attitudes, we will remain a slave to our old habits.*

Capture the Power of Your Emotions

The critical importance of experiencing a personal tipping point cannot be overstated. The tipping point, disguised as a defeat, tragedy or misfortune is actually a *gift* - if you are ready to do something positive. It is a unique opportunity to align your body and mind into an extremely powerful force.

Jump on this opportunity!

Note: Jealousy and envy are not necessarily desirable emotions but are normal to the human condition and can be used by you to great advantage. They are simply a signal telling you that you want something more out of life than what you have right now. Give yourself the opportunity to get it!

Don't bury your emotions or let them consume your life in a negative downward spiral. The trick is to use these incredibly powerful feelings and channel them into positive thoughts and actions that will transform your life forever.

Is the glass half full? Bingo, you got it baby! *Attitude...*

This is your time, right now. This is the place. It is your destiny to get this done and create an extraordinary life full of love, joy and accomplishment. Your **Big Dream** is waiting for you. All you have to do is *believe* it's your turn, *believe* you deserve it and *believe* that nothing will stop you.

Are you feeling it - are you ready?

Ready, Fire, Aim – You're Not Ready Yet
No, you're not quite ready yet. You're well on your way, but there are a few more hoops to pass through to ensure your success.

Right now, you've got one or more of these very negative thoughts, feelings and emotions about yourself and about others that are flowing through your veins - anger, fear, hurt, sadness, jealousy or envy.

Your next step is the most critical in the *Weight Loss for Wimps*™ process. And that is to transform these very real and important negative emotions into something very, very positive:

A white hot, forward looking, unstoppable desire and vision of yourself as the healthy, sexy, thin person you will become.

This will be our focus in the next chapter.

Weight Loss for Wimps ™
Success Step Two

Attitude: I have experienced an unpleasant tipping point in my life. I have decided that I <u>want</u> to resolve my weight issue <u>now</u>.

The glass is half full, not half empty.

Skills: I will allow myself to feel these negative emotions, recognizing that they are important and a necessary part of the process.

I will see my tipping point situation as a unique *opportunity* and a "gift" for achieving health, happiness and incredible weight loss success.

Action: Spend at least 30 minutes in quiet reflection, writing down a brief description of your tipping point(s) and noting the key negative emotions that you are feeling about it.

Think about <u>you</u>, not about others. Start thinking more about the present and your future, and less about your past. The eyes are on the **FRONT** of your head!

<u>Important Notes:</u>
If you feel that you have *not* yet experienced a critical tipping point in your life… that's ok. It may mean you are fairly satisfied with your situation and not quite ready to tackle your weight issue *at this time*.

You will know when it happens and you will know when it's time to do something positive about it. The last thing you want to do is force yourself to do something because you *think* you "should." It just won't work until you and your body decide that it's something you passionately <u>*want*</u> to do.

If your tipping point and weight issue are related to a <u>traumatic</u> incident i.e. rape, sexual abuse or physical abuse, please seek professional medical help. The techniques herein may help but are not intended as a substitute for professional guidance.

CHAPTER THREE

LIFESTYLE BREAKOUT™
THE CORNERSTONE STRATEGY

OVERVIEW OF THE Lifestyle Breakout™ Strategy

This chapter presents what I call the Lifestyle Breakout™ Strategy. It is the cornerstone of the *Weight Loss for Wimps™ System* because it is here, through proper implementation of this process, that you will develop the ***magical mindset mojo power*** to conquer your obesity issue forever.

Your mind is the most powerful organ in your body and the most powerful tool at your disposal for creating a healthy, slim figure and a healthy, pleasurable lifestyle. The connection between your mind and the health of your body is scientifically irrefutable.

Research over the past 10 years has clearly demonstrated the physiological effects of using the centuries old placebo to effectively treat a wide variety of diseases (see Scientific American, February, 2009 for a good summary).

The placebo effect aside, evidence indicates that at least 75% of people who receive medical treatment show improvement simply because they *believe* the treatment will work.

Don't worry - I'm not going to take you into a world of psycho-babble, self-hypnosis or affirmations. These techniques may have benefits but they're not my area of expertise. I'm going to share with you solid, down-to-earth thought processes that worked for me and have worked for my weight loss mentoring clients.

The goal of the *Lifestyle Breakout™ Strategy* is simply this:

"Develop your Mindset Mojo in order to take those negative emotions from your tipping point experience and use them to create an unstoppable weight loss mindset to achieve your **Big Dream**.*"*

To accomplish this, let's work together through the following process:

1. Acknowledge the self-imposed constraints of the status quo
2. Discover the "real reason" you want to lose weight and become thin

3. Imagine, in specific detail, your *Big Dream*
4. Sell yourself on the *Big Dream*

Simple goal, challenging process. Let's get going!

1. The Status Quo (Wimpdom) Is Not Your Friend

As humans, one of our greatest failures is to consistently accept our current situation as inevitable... We tell ourselves stories that justify our lives and wimpy behaviors. For example:

Story: "I'm overweight because my mother was overweight and fed us bad food as kids. Plus, I inherited a slow metabolism."

Reality: "I'm overweight because I eat too much of the wrong foods and never exercise."

The truth is, we tend to stay in our comfort zone because it is the easiest thing to do. It is the path of least resistance. No additional effort is required. We just keep doing whatever it is we're doing and dreaming about how things *should* have been different, *could* have been different "...if only..." but we never find the motivation to actually *do* anything about it. This is what we wimps do!

The first step in the Lifestyle Breakout™ Strategy is to affirmatively admit to ourselves that the way things are, the status quo, is **unacceptable**. Your current habits, current view of yourself and your future prospects are self-imposed limitations. You created this box, this cocoon because it's a great story you've told yourself… "poor me…"

If your "comfort zone" includes feelings of insecurity, self-doubt, anger, fear about your future, low self-esteem, or lack of self confidence then it's time to do something about it. And the best place to start is by regaining your health and losing *all* of your excess weight.

You could make many changes in your life - new job, new boyfriend, move to a different town, earn your degree, but there is *nothing* that will match the benefits of changing your lifestyle habits to achieve your perfect weight and good health. Nothing.

Acknowledge the past, acknowledge the present and vow to create your own future.

2. Discover the REAL Reason You Want to Be Thin

The incident or series of incidents that caused your tipping point may have no direct connection to the real reason you want to lose weight.

The purpose of this step is to dig deep and discover the real reason you want to be thin. Do not skim over this - spend an hour or two in brutally honest self-reflection. Keep asking yourself <u>why</u>?

In my own case, I wanted to get thin for health reasons. Many people have mild to serious health issues, so let's go through a brief self-reflection example.

"<u>Why</u> do you want to lose weight and become thin?"

"My health is getting worse and I keep getting heavier."

"<u>Why</u> is your health getting worse and <u>Why</u> are you gaining weight?"

"I've got heart disease, Type 2 diabetes, high blood pressure and my knees are in bad shape. I guess I'm gaining more weight because I'm not exercising."

"<u>Why</u> are you not eating healthy foods and getting at least some exercise?"

"Well…I love certain foods and I have trouble with the idea of giving them up."

"You know that losing all your excess weight and eating healthy, clean food can stop or even reverse your heart disease, diabetes and high blood pressure. <u>Why</u> isn't that more important than "giving up a few favorite foods?"

"It *is* more important. I want to see my kids' graduate from college, get married and I'd like to travel to Kenya to photograph the wildebeest migration in the Masai Mara Reserve. It's something I've dreamed about all my life. I'm not healthy enough to make the trip right now…"

"<u>Why</u> have you just given up on the idea? You know with a few lifestyle changes, it's within your reach?"

For another example, let's say you decide you want to be thin "because I want to be hot and sexy."

Ok, nothing wrong with that. For some, that reason may be a bit too superficial, but who cares! If that's what works for you, let's work with it…

"<u>Why</u> do you want to become hot and sexy?"

"Well, I think it would be cool to have an attractive body."

"<u>Why</u> is having an attractive body important to you?"

"Well, if I had a nice thin body, I could attract a nice husband."

"<u>Why</u> is that important to you?"

"I've never had a serious relationship. I'd like to fall in love and have a family."

"Have you had a serious relationship in the past?"

"I don't get asked out much. In fact, I hardly ever get asked out."

"WHY do you think that is the case?"

"I've been overweight since I was a teenager. I had a boyfriend (or husband) for a while, but he dumped me."

"<u>Why</u> did he dump you?"

"Probably because I was fat and needy, angry, demanding, insecure… (fill in your story)"

Keep going with this self-reflection process. It will likely bring to the surface some very intense feelings of hurt, disappointment and fear. Think about your self-image - how you view yourself in the world and how you compare yourself to others. Think about your future; three years from now; seven years from now…

If you feel like crying… cry! And cry some more. It's an important and healthy part of the self discovery process. You need to understand, at a deep emotional level, how being overweight *really* affects your daily life. How it affects your personality, your outlook on the future - everything.

Maybe your primary motivation is revenge… yeah, that can work too! Imagine the look on your ex's face!

Keep searching, keep questioning yourself, keep asking why. Now, start thinking about how your life would change if you were at your ideal weight. How would you feel about yourself… how would you feel walking into the room at your class reunion?

You'll know when you discover the real reason why you want to be thin and healthy, because it is something you are willing to <u>fight for</u> with everything you have inside your mind. ***It is the single most important benefit you will gain by reaching your perfect weight.***

You've begun the process of transforming those gut-wrenching, negative emotions that started with your tipping point, into something far more powerful.

3. Imagine You Strutting Your Stuff – The Big Dream
Now comes the fun part of the *Lifestyle Breakout™* process - developing a crystal clear vision of your **Big Dream!**

You will never rise above the way you visualize yourself, so think healthy, think thin, and **Dream Big!**

Imagine you at your perfect weight. The new clothes you will be wearing. The new hairstyle you've selected. The classy new shoes, the confidence you will carry as you approach the podium to speak, or as you walk down the aisle at the wedding.

We think in pictures, so think in bright, exciting colors and see yourself like you've never seen yourself before interacting with real people in your life, introducing yourself to someone new, having lunch with so-and-so, going to the new job interview. Imagine every detail of how you will look, and also how you will feel as you go about your day in your new, healthy body.

Use your imagination to create a new story about yourself. A healthy, empowered vision of yourself having reached your perfect weight. This new story about you will create new thought patterns and eventually new, positive behaviors.

Capture in your mind the new confidence you have in yourself. Visualize yourself making great decisions as you go out to your favorite restaurant with your spouse, date or loved ones. Imagine going to the grocery store or farmer's market and selecting healthy foods and then going home to prepare a fantastic meal for your family.

Fantasies are the fuel of life, so let your imagination go wild and put yourself in a variety of situations and scenarios.

Imagine you… strutting your stuff…

Imagine you… cool, articulate, charming, self confident…

Imagine you… landing that big promotion or important client…

Imagine you… holding that newborn baby…

Imagine you… shooting hoops or water skiing…

Imagine you… fitting into those size four jeans…

Imagine you… at the beach in your new bikini…

Did you come up with a killer scenario that is absolutely your favorite vision of yourself in the future? Does it include the *real reason* you want to be thin? Is it the one that really gets your emotions flowing, your passions "white-hot"?

Revisit and re-think that scenario in great detail. That's your keeper - that's your **_Big Dream_**. It is this vision of yourself that you want to play over and over in your mind on a daily basis, as you struggle at times during your weight loss process to stay on track.

It is this "white-hot" vision of yourself that will carry the day when your mental enemies (excuses, emotional eating, stress, hunger) gang up on you and want you to quit.

Now you've got the **Big Dream** firmly planted in your brain. You've got a new life to live; in the future you create for yourself.

In addition to achieving your **Big Dream**, you will get some "side benefits" that you may not even anticipate. In my own case, here are just a few:

- Ability to play softball again, after 20 years of inactivity
- Having friends that I haven't seen in a while say, "Wow! You look 15 years younger… at least!"

- Seeing a high school friend who said, "Is that really you? You look like a basketball player instead of the big football lineman!"
- Having my doctor say, "Your blood measurements are perfect, and you did 13 minutes on the stress test. That's athlete level conditioning!"

4. Believe in the Big Dream

Is your **Big Dream** really possible? Of course it is. If you believe it - it will happen.

The most important question you must ask yourself right now...

Why Not Me?"

What you believe will determine what you will achieve. Talk to yourself at the emotional level. Sell yourself on your **Big Dream**. This is the most important goal you must achieve in your life right now.

Regardless of your past, your present circumstances, your sex or your age, you deserve to be healthy, sexy, happy and thin. It's your turn. Do you want it bad enough to do the work?

Key Concept: The most powerful way to sell your **Big Dream** to yourself is to write it down in your journal. This simple technique further develops your **mindset mojo thought process** and reinforces the *Lifestyle Breakout™ Strategy* by a factor of 10 - just do it and you will see!

You now have the power, the juice, and the mojo to solve your obesity puzzle once and for all. In the next chapter, you will learn how to transform your **Big Dream** into action with a laser focused intensity that will make you truly unstoppable!

**Weight Loss for Wimps™
Success Step Three**

> **Attitude**: I realize that the status quo – my habits, behaviors, the way I view myself, the way I view my future – is wimpy and unacceptable
>
> I take full responsibility for creating my own future
>
> **Skills**: I will be brutally honest with myself to discover the real reason I want to be thin – the single most important benefit to me

I will use my imagination to create an exciting, vivid vision of myself at my perfect weight. This will be my **Big Dream**.

<u>**Action**</u>: Take notes in your daily journal as you work through the <u>why</u> questions to select your biggest benefit of getting thin

Use your journal to write down the specific details of your **Big Dream**. Include feelings of empowerment, self confidence, energy and happiness. This will solidify your belief and help to make it become a reality.

CHAPTER FOUR

MAKING <u>YOU</u> PRIORITY NUMBER ONE

HAVE YOU EVER gone to a seminar or purchased a self-help book, gotten all excited, enthusiastic, pumped up... and then within hours or a couple of days, finding yourself slowly drifting back to your daily routine... promising yourself you will get started "soon"?

This chapter is designed to eliminate that problem...at least as it applies to the *Weight Loss for Wimps™ System*.

After the Dog, Honey, Of Course You're Number One

Just joking, of course. Your husband/wife wouldn't really say that to you, right? But, he/she might act like that at times. After all, he/she' is busy with the kids, job, volunteer work, golf, yard work... he/she has got his/her life to live too.

The point is, the only person who can make you, your health, and your weight loss goal the number one priority in your life is <u>you</u>.

That was the huge advantage and an "a-ha!" moment for me when I went to weight loss camp for three weeks. I was 100% focused on my health, 24/7.

But most people don't have the time (or money) available to go to a weight loss camp. And besides, when you get back to real life after going to camp, then what?

You and only you can make it happen by taking full responsibility and making healthy eating, exercise, and weight loss the number one priority in your life. Period.

Give Yourself Permission To Be Number One
For many of us, giving ourselves permission to be priority #1 is very difficult. We feel very guilty or sometimes, we use it as an excuse. Naturally, mothers tend to put their families first, and men generally put their jobs first (just my observation, not necessarily applicable to you).

But, if you are going to achieve the **Big Dream**, if you have the passion to finally get your health and weight under control, you <u>must</u> make this mindset shift. At least for 6 months or so while you are beating down your bad habits and implementing new, healthy ones.

84

That means your job, your spouse, and yes even your kids, must be put on the back burner, figuratively speaking. It doesn't mean you ignore these important aspects of your life. It just means that you devote your mental and physical energy to your health <u>first</u>, and take care of the other people and activities that you are responsible for <u>second</u>. ***Realize that this is emotional maturity, not selfishness.***

Sure, it's going to mean some changes in your daily routine that others may notice…

- You may decide to go to bed an hour earlier to get up an hour earlier to exercise and have a healthy breakfast
- You may spend time every Sunday preparing your lunches for the coming week
- You may decide to limit your TV to one hour a day and spend more time outside playing with your kids
- You may decide to pass on the Friday after work drinks with your co-workers
- You may decide to go to the gym or play racquetball during your lunch hour or right after work
- You may decide to sign up for kick-boxing classes on Tuesday nights

- You may decide to go for a fifteen minute walk twice a day during your breaks
- You may decide to quit buying any soda, cola or other soft drinks (you think the kids will notice?)
- You may decide to quit drinking any beer and switch to red wine instead
- You may decide to give up, or at least suspend, some activities to give yourself more time to focus on your health

Whatever you decide, things are going to change in your life. You are going to take control and ***give yourself permission*** to make <u>*you priority number one*</u>.

The Healthy Obsession – All Day, Every Day
For the next six months (at least), your health, your weight loss goal, your **Big Dream** must become your *healthy obsession*. That means you think about it first thing when you wake up in the morning, periodically throughout the day and think about it as you close your eyes to go to sleep at night… all day, every day.

This is absolutely necessary to fight off the bad habit demons that will try constantly to derail your efforts. And it's necessary so that you will remain focused like a laser beam on your goal, your **Big Dream** and your health. It is only through constant and sustained *focus* that you will come out a winner.

Every day you will be faced with over 200 food choices that you have to deal with, in the moment, and make a decision (based on research by Dr. Brian Wansink, Cornell University, 2007).

- "Do I grab that donut in the break room or just a cup of coffee?"

- "Do I eat a healthy meal at home before I go to the cocktail party or eat the junk food I know they will be serving?"

- "Do I brown bag a healthy lunch today or hit Burger King around the corner from the office?"

- "Do I put a bottle of water and some raisins or nuts in my purse before going to the movies or go for the buttered popcorn and Coke?"

- "Do I continue buying snacks out of the vending machines or think ahead and bring some sliced fruit and veggies to work?"

Not to mention choices about physical exercise...

- "Do I get my butt out of bed and go exercise, or do I pull the covers up and go back to sleep for a little while longer?"

- "Do I work late today (to look good to my boss) or hit the gym right after work, as promised?"

All day, every day you keep your crystal clear vision of your **Big Dream** front and center in your thoughts, and you consistently ask yourself...

"Does this move me closer to my goal?"

And then you smile and pat yourself on the back for making the right decision.

You're not "toughing it out," or "making the sacrifice" or "sucking it up"... you're taking action, changing your lifestyle permanently, moving towards your **Big Dream**, loving yourself, feeling more confident; and it feels - G-R-E-A-T!

You've got the *mindset mojo,* the power and are now well on your way to becoming an unstoppable force in pursuit of your health, happiness and your **Big Dream**.

The next step in our planning process is setting your weight loss goal. We'll tackle that in the next chapter.

Weight Loss for Wimps™
Success Step Four

> Attitude: I give myself permission to make my health and weight loss goal priority number one in my life.
>
> I am developing a healthy obsession about creating a mindset and lifestyle that will allow me to achieve my **Big Dream**
>
> Skills: All day, every day I will reflect on the vision of my **Big Dream**
>
> As I make my daily decisions on food choices and exercise, I will always ask

myself, "*Does this move me closer to my goal or not?*"

Action: In your personal journal, write down specific changes you will commit to making, in your daily routine, to accommodate your new lifestyle.

Include a list of activities that you will eliminate, suspend or delegate to others to give you more time to focus on tasks related to your health and wellness.

Create a list of *new* activities that you want to do such as learning healthy meal preparation, going to the gym, riding your bicycle, taking a brisk walk, or shopping at the farmer's market.

CHAPTER FIVE

SETTING YOUR WEIGHT LOSS GOAL

SETTING A WEIGHT LOSS goal is an important component of the *Weight Loss for Wimps*™ process. You need a specific goal set in advance, so that you can monitor your progress and make any necessary adjustments along the way.

You need to know where you're going so you can celebrate when you arrive!

When Twenty Pounds Isn't Good Enough
When I started my last (and final) weight loss journey, I didn't set a goal in advance. In my typical fashion, I just told myself, "I need to lose some weight." Within a month or so of being a tough guy (like how long can you hold your breath underwater?), I had lost 20 lbs.

That was good. I was starting to feel a little better and my clothes sure fit much better. On the surface, things were looking much brighter.

The problem was, I was fighting it every step of the way and I certainly had no plan and no weight loss objective in mind. And sure enough,

I started cheating regularly, patting myself on the back with false bravado, and began packing the lbs back on.

Twenty lbs was a good start, but when you need to lose 100 lbs to reach your perfect weight, that's all it is, a good start.

Until I had my breakthrough "white hot" moment with clarity of vision on what I really wanted to achieve (described earlier), I was like a sailboat drifting at sea; I'd get a little wind for a while but had no course to sail and no final destination in mind.

That's when I made the decision to get healthy once and for all, and reduce down to my "perfect weight."

What's Your Perfect Weight?
The issue of deciding what your "perfect weight" should be can get a little confusing and even controversial, depending on your source of information. I like to keep things simple so I recommend you use the Body Mass Index (BMI) calculator and standard weight ranges based on the BMI. This methodology is used and accepted by the premiere health organizations worldwide.

BMI is simply a calculation of body fatness, based on a person's height and weight. Although the mathematical formula used is relatively simple, the results have shown to have a very high correlation to more precise measurements such as caliper skin fold thickness and underwater weighing (among others).

The US Center for Disease Control (CDC) has a handy BMI calculator on their website, which you can access here (for adults 20 years old and older; note there is also a different calculator for children and teenagers):
http://tinyurl.com/b53foz
The standard weight status categories associated with BMI ranges for adults are shown in the following table:

BMI	Weight Status
Below 18.5	Underweight
18.5 – 24.9	Normal
25.0 – 29.9	Overweight
30.0 and Above	Obese

What is a healthy weight for you?

There are a variety of online calculators; some include age, sex in addition to the standard height. To make things simple, I recommend going to the Weight Watchers® calculator here: http://www.weightwatchers.com/health/asm/cal c_healthyweight.aspx

Are you shocked? Fearful? Anxious?

Don't be. Just relax because getting to your perfect weight will be much easier than you think. You've got the *Lifestyle Breakout*™ system on your side, which you've never had before. And in the coming chapters you will be learning some very specific techniques for dealing with your mental enemies and strategies for eating healthy and exercising properly.

For now, let's just agree that your weight loss goal will be the weight that is no higher than the BMI=25 for your height.

Why am I pushing you so hard?

Because overwhelming medical evidence is clear that you are at a much higher risk of serious disease (heart disease, diabetes, stroke, osteoarthritis and some cancers) if you fit into the overweight or obesity ranges.

I know that selling you on the idea of prevention is much harder than selling you a cure. But trust me, once you have any of these diseases, your life will change in ways that you cannot even imagine.

And if you do have any of these diseases, your life could improve dramatically and possibly even reverse your condition if you start eating healthy and get your weight down to where it should be.

Notwithstanding the medical advantages, how about other aspects of your Big Dream? And the "side benefits?" Imagine you, strutting your stuff, at your perfect weight!

All In – Go For the Gold and an Extraordinary Life

Do you play Texas Hold 'em or ever watch championship poker on TV?

I love to see it when a player goes "all in."

That means he or she bets their entire stash of chips - going for broke, going after the big pot.

There are times in life that you should put it all on the line. This is one of those times.

Why settle for mediocrity when with a little more effort you can go for gold and create an extraordinary life and lifestyle for yourself?

I want you to go "all in."

Break It Down – One Month At A Time

Now that you have your big picture goal, you need to break it down into small increments. For this, I suggest setting a monthly weight loss goal of about 10 lbs, for most people.

Why 10 lbs a month?

It's comfortable. It's realistic. It's healthy. It's obtainable.

I'm sure you want to lose more weight, much faster. That's human nature... instant gratification, right?

You can certainly do that. In fact it's easy... just reduce your caloric intake more and increase the time and intensity of your exercise. That will work for a while...

The problem with shooting for rapid weight loss is that you will, in short order; put your body into "survival mode." That means your body will slow your metabolism down significantly (regardless of your exercise amount) as it tries to conserve fat and energy. It also triggers hormonal changes that actually cause you to crave food and stimulates food-seeking behaviors and even start metabolizing muscle tissue… not a good thing! Besides, you don't want to be hungry all the time!

Certainly, you need to reduce your caloric intake to a level below your food input otherwise you can't lose weight. The trick is to do it modestly, so your survival mode is not triggered. There are several strategies to do this and we'll discuss that more fully in Part Three.

The main idea here is to get over the quick weight loss mindset. Think strategically and long term. That means breaking the yo-yo diet cycle, learning to eat plenty of great tasting, nutritious whole foods that will satisfy your hunger and heal your body.

You didn't gain the weight overnight so don't expect to lose it overnight. Setting a goal of 10 lbs a month or 2-3 lbs a week is optimal if you have 25+ lbs to lose. It's easy to monitor on a weekly basis and then you make adjustments to your intake and exercise, as needed to keep you on track.

Just imagine yourself 60 lbs lighter in six short months… awesome!

Your momentum is building and with the tools and tactics you will be learning next, you will have the wind at your back.

**Weight Loss for Wimps™
Success Step Five**

Attitude: I am going to solve my weight issue once and for all

I am going "all in" to improve my health, achieve my **Big Dream** and create an extraordinary life

Skills: I will use the CDC (or similar) website to calculate my current BMI

I will use the Weight Watchers® or similar calculator to determine my long-term perfect weight goal

My short-term weight loss goal will be approximately 10 lbs per month

Action: Take a couple of photos of yourself now. Later on, you'll look at them and feel proud and amazed at your transformation.

Record your current height and weight, your starting BMI and your perfect weight goal in your daily journal.

Make a chart to record your weekly/monthly progress. Include other key measurement such as waist, thighs, and arms. You may also want to record your % weight lost on a monthly basis. This is calculated as follows: lbs lost over the month divided by starting weight at beginning of the month, times 100.

Example of Percentage Weight Loss Calculation:

Starting weight at beginning of month: 184 lbs
Weight at end of month: <u>174</u> lbs
Lbs lost: 10 lbs

10 lbs divided by 184 lbs = 0.05 X 100 = 5% weight loss

CHAPTER SIX

YOU'VE GOT POWERFUL OBSTACLES: KNOWING YOUR ENEMIES

CHALK TALK – The Big Picture
Before we dive in to discussing our common enemies, let's review the big picture about where we are in the *Weight Loss for Wimps*™ process and where we're going.

I like to use a sports analogy because most people have some familiarity (if not a burning passion) for a team sport – soccer, baseball, football, basketball, etc. Let's say I'm the coach and I've recruited you to play on my football team.

My basic coaching philosophy is this:

"Plan every battle and win it twice... once in your mind and then on the field."

We've got a big game coming up next week and my job is to get you prepared to play your best. One of the tools I use to get you ready is a classroom "chalk talk."

On the blackboard, I draw up plays, defensive strategies, and have extensive discussions about our opponent. I'll talk about their strengths and weaknesses, about what it means to win this game, and our overall strategies. We'll look at game films to study the opposing teams' best plays and identify their best players.

Then, we'll develop specific how-to tactics. We'll visualize on the blackboard and in our minds each and every move they will make (anticipation) and every move we will make on the playing field in order to defeat them.

We then go to the practice field and we'll practice our moves until they are well rehearsed, *in advance*.

On game day, we're ready. It's time for action and implementation of our strategy and specific tactics.

Let's get it on!

If you execute, as planned, you will win most of the battles and rack up the most points - ***Game Over***.

The Big Four Bad Boys
You already know that the deck is stacked against you in making this dramatic lifestyle change to eating healthy, exercising properly and losing weight. As mentioned previously, 90% of people ultimately fail.

I mention this again only to emphasize the importance of preparing your mind to win. You *will* be among the elite 10% crowd because you *will* be prepared to fight the daily battles that will be raging in your mind and body as you start on this exciting adventure (it gets much easier over time).

The vast majority of people never give any serious thought to preparation when they start a weight loss program or "diet." And that is why the majority of people fail.

Your mind and body are in their "comfort zone" at the beginning and would prefer to stay there... it's easy... the path of least resistance.

In order to win these battles, you need to know who your enemies are and how to defeat them consistently.

Let's begin by meeting the major players on the other team who will operate behind the scenes to create obstacles, hoping you will give up and return to your normal, wimp lifestyle, with your tail between your legs.

By way of introduction, here are the bad boys that are out to defeat you:

- Excuses
- Emotional Eating
- Stress
- Physical Hunger

These are powerful, very powerful and very resourceful enemies. Going up against them is like playing in the Super Bowl or World Cup. Preparation is key. I'll get you trained on how to defeat these bullies in the coming chapters.

Can You Win Every Battle?
Theoretically, yes - you can win every battle, every day.

Realistically, no - we are all human and therefore imperfect. It would be unrealistic and unreasonable to set that kind of a standard for yourself.

Forgive yourself right now, in advance!

There will be days, moments, instances where everything goes out the window and you blow it - you cheat on your eating program and or your exercise routine. Like everything else in the *Weight Loss for Wimps™* program, expect it, plan on it and learn to work through it.

How to Cheat Successfully: Introducing the *No Fear™* Cheating Technique

It's a little strange, putting "cheat" and "successfully" in the same sentence, but why not? It's going to happen so let's not make a big deal out of it. It's not the end of the world!

Naturally, you want to shoot for 100% compliance, 100% of the time. You will reach your goal and reap the **Big Dream** benefits much faster. But 90%-95% is more realistic. When you do cheat, understand that it simply means that you slow down the process a bit. That said; let's learn how to do it with *gusto* and *joy*.

First, let me make a confession. I've cheated on occasion throughout my 88 lb weight loss journey. And you will too.

Here is the cheating system that I have developed and found to be most effective in limiting the damage. I call it the "*No Fear*™ Cheating Technique"

- **N**o bingeing allowed. Always plan your cheating in advance. This can be anything from an hour or two or a day or two. The main thing is to break the cycle of "sudden, uncontrollable urges" that you may have had in the past. These are related to emotional eating which will be detailed in Chapter 8.

- **O**nly allow yourself a few bites of the "forbidden food"; don't pig out on the entire bag of chips or eat the entire container of ice cream.

- **F**orgive yourself in advance; don't beat yourself up, feel worthless, angry, or upset. Understand it's part of the process of learning to eat healthy

- **E**njoy every bite, savor the flavor explosion in your mouth and concentrate on what you are eating. Guiltlessly.

- **A**sk yourself, after you're finished
  …"Did it taste as good as I expected?
  Did it satisfy my lust for that particular
  food?"

- **R**evert back to your healthy eating
  program…*immediately*…not next week.
  Make an immediate commitment to
  yourself to 100% compliance.

What I found is that over time, the desire to
cheat diminishes significantly and that the
pleasure derived from eating the "forbidden
food" also diminishes significantly.

This is going to sound strange but trust me, it's
true - the cravings I now get on occasion are for
certain healthy foods that I haven't eaten in a
while, like out of season fruit or vegetables.

Plan, anticipate and execute the *No Fear*™
cheating technique and you will soon be craving
a mango instead of a Big Mac! Unbelievable to
you now, but true. It works.

Let's get going on learning specific tactics for
dealing with the Bad Boys. In the next chapter,
we'll start with Wimpy Excuses.

**Weight Loss for Wimps™
Success Step Six**

Attitude: I know the odds are against me and I've failed before. But this time is different because I'm thinking about my enemies and making plans to defeat them, *in advance*.

I am going to Anticipate, Plan and Execute

Skills: I have learned how to cheat successfully. As needed, I will implement the *No Fear™* cheating technique and use this skill with joy and without guilt. I understand this is part of the process of becoming healthy and thin.

When a cheating event occurs, I will *immediately* get back on my healthy eating program…with a smile on my face!

Action: Record in your daily journal the *No Fear™* cheating technique. Memorize the sequence so it will always be with you when needed.

Think about your current eating habits and patterns. Make notes in your journal about particular events, locations, situations or people that in retrospect, seem to trigger an overeating reaction in you. These are areas you need to work on.

PART TWO

TOOLS AND TACTICS
FOR
WINNING EVERY BATTLE

CHAPTER SEVEN

TACTICS FOR DEALING WITH
WIMPY EXCUSES

EXCUSES ARE A Dime a Dozen
Excuses can best be described as the little stories we tell ourselves (and others) to justify the status quo and explain why we *can't* do something (like eating healthy or exercising regularly). They are insidious little creatures in our mind that typically start out as a single thought and then morph and multiply like rabbits as we come up with better ones. Ultimately, we find one that works well for us and then stick with it until challenged.

I've created and used many, many excuses over the years. How about you? See if you can spot your favorite excuse - as you will see, these are all very, very *Wimpy*!

Going on a diet, eating healthy, losing weight, or exercising won't work for me because...

- "I'm big boned..."
- "I travel a lot..."
- "I'm too busy with my kids and job..."
- "My metabolism is too slow..."

- "I have so much to lose and it will take too long…"
- "I love good food and can't give it up…"
- "Counting calories is too hard…"
- "I can't cook…"
- "I don't have any willpower…"
- "It runs in the family so I inherited it…"
- "I have too many business trips, social obligations…"
- "My husband and kids insist I feed them what they like…"
- "Healthy food costs too much…"
- "I'm going on vacation in two weeks so I'll start after that…"
- "I'm not an athlete so I can't work out or go to the gym…"
- "My friends eat junk food so it's hard for me…"
- "I hate to exercise because it makes me hungry…"
- "I blew it today, so I'll get started again next Monday…"
- "I'll just sleep for a few minutes longer…"

The list of excuses is actually without limits, left only to your imagination. If you read through the list slowly and carefully a couple of times, you'll see that there are easy solutions to each one. It's all about developing your **mindset mojo** and forming new thought patterns.

There are two excuses in particular that I want to address first, because they are potential deal stoppers. They are especially insidious, tricky and deceitful…

"I know I'm overweight, but I'm really happy just the way I am."

If this describes you, I'm very happy for you. Every person on this earth deserves to be happy and live a full, healthy life. But my question is, *"If this is really true, why are you reading this book?"*

In my experience, I have yet to meet someone who is significantly overweight and truly happy about it. I'm sure there are people who are, I just haven't met any.

Maybe you are relatively young, have a life partner and are not experiencing any serious health problems. But it is highly likely that you will at some point, more likely sooner than later. And it's totally preventable if you take action now.

Stop. Go someplace quiet. Close your eyes and be brutally honest with yourself. You know this excuse is wrong…dead wrong. Give it up, now. Join with us on this life changing journey that you will never, ever regret.

"I've tried many diets and I'm afraid to try again and fail."

This one is different because it indicates that you are not happy at your current weight and that you really would like to do something about it. That's the good news, but…

It's a very dangerous "excuse" on a couple of levels. First and most importantly it signals that you have been using this excuse to just *give up*. That, of course, leads to doing nothing and continuing along the path of mediocrity and unhappiness. If you've read this far in the book, hopefully you are no longer willing to just give up.

Fear of failure is actually an illusion in that people are not really "afraid to fail" (who hasn't failed on a diet?), they are just fearful that they *don't know how to succeed*. The *Weight Loss for Wimps*™ system should remove that fear forever. You will know how to succeed and you will be motivated to do the necessary work to reach your goal.

Dead on Arrival Excuses

Let's go back to our list of excuses and briefly address each one:

- *"I'm big boned..."*
  I'm not exactly sure what big boned is...does someone actually measure bone size? You may have a big body but it has nothing to do with the size of your bones. Do all people who are at normal weight have "small bones"? I don't think so.

- *"I travel a lot..."*
  That's great, I'm happy for you. Other people are envious that you get to travel and they don't. What does that have to do with eating healthy? Famous movie stars, models, athletes, business executives, airline pilots, military personnel and TV media personalities all over the world travel a lot too. Most of them are thin and healthy. What are they doing differently that you're not?

- *"I'm too busy with my kids and job..."*

I'm sure you are very busy. Probably too busy. What can you quit doing to give yourself more time to devote to your health? Make yourself <u>priority number one,</u> for at least six months. You deserve this chance to build a healthy lifestyle. By the way, thin people are busy too - what are they doing differently?

- *"My metabolism is too slow..."*
  It is possible that you might have an under active thyroid condition (hypothyroidism) and if you suspect that, get it checked by a physician; it can be easily treated. However, your resting metabolic rate can be significantly increased by activity (walking, swimming), adding lean muscle tissue (resistance training) and by proper nutrition (energy stabilizing food). In other words, if it's slow, speed it up!

- *"I have so much to lose and it will take too long..."*
  This one is counter-intuitive and defies logic. Nevertheless, the mindset should be, *I've got a lot to lose, so let's get going!* The more you have to lose, the more you will lose particularly during the early stages of your program. Some

115

of the Biggest Loser folks have lost 22 lbs in a week!

- *"I love good food and can't give it up..."*
  On any healthy, sensible, nutritious eating program, there are certain foods that you *will* have to give up. These fall into the "cut the crap" category and include sugar, processed foods i.e. fake foods, chips, sodas, white flour and rice, and white breads (more details in Part Three). That leaves a huge variety of "good food" with which to make delicious meals.

- *"Counting calories is too hard..."*
  Calorie counting is not really hard, it's just a little time consuming. I don't like it either and generally don't do it myself. There are many good eating programs that don't require it; the South Beach Diet® comes to mind, for example. However, it is important that you learn to read food labels and become intimately familiar with the calorie content and nutritional values of the foods you eat. By taking this step, you can better control your caloric intake

without having to add columns of numbers.

- *"I can't cook…"*
  I can barely boil water so I am sympathetic to this one. Fortunately for me, I have a spouse who is a very talented cook who also enjoys researching recipes and experimenting with different dishes. Without a cook in the house, you have two options; exert a little effort and learn to cook a few good meals that you like; or buy your meals outside the home. Grocery store deli's often have great salad and soup bars and there are many restaurants where you can order fabulous healthy meals (if you choose carefully).

- *"I don't have any willpower…"*
  Willpower is not the answer to a successful lifestyle change. The key is adopting the entire *Lifestyle Breakout*™ set of attitudes, skills and knowledge. Your imagination and **Big Dream** will provide you with the self discipline to get through the tough moments that will inevitably come.

- *"It runs in the family so I inherited it…"*
  This is a very convenient excuse but just doesn't cut it. Researchers have found that genetics only accounts for *up to* 25% of a person's weight; that means *at least* 75% of your weight issue can be controlled by your eating and exercise behaviors. Here's an interesting clue for animal lovers - studies show that many overweight families have pets that are also overweight. Why do you suppose that is the case? The dog sure doesn't have your genes!

- *"I have too many business trips, social obligations…"*
  Business travel was discussed above. Social obligations (cocktail parties, dinners, company picnics, business lunches, weddings, etc.) are an important part of many people's lives. These are events that you should look forward to attending. And they offer you a great opportunity to demonstrate to yourself and others that you know how to eat healthy and how to control your impulses. You can't '*not go*' to these events just because you've changed your eating habits. Use them to reinforce your new, good habits. *(Tip – eat a healthy*

snack before you go if you're worried about what will be served.)

- *"My husband and kids insist I feed them what they like…"*
  You have two choices on this one: (a) you can be a short order cook and feed everyone exactly what they want. Or, (b) you can have a family meeting, seek their assistance and work towards getting the entire family to eat healthy. The obvious choice is b but either way, <u>you</u> still control what goes in your mouth. You may need to get tough and use the old comedian Buddy Hackett's line…"You have two choices: take it or leave it!"

- *"Healthy food costs too much…"*
  Yes, it is true that some fruits, vegetables, fish, meat, nuts, whole grain breads and pastas are a bit more expensive, particularly when buying organic. However, most of these additional costs are almost completely offset when you quit buying all of the "cheaper" processed fake foods. It's amazing how all the chips, cookies, ice cream, cakes, catsup, mayonnaise, sausage, hotdogs, beer, and candy add

119

up to some serious bucks at the checkout counter.

- *"I'm going on vacation in two weeks so I'll start after that..."*
Why not start right now? In two weeks, you'll have most of your new style of eating down so you can continue on with it during your vacation. Is it written somewhere that you must pig out while you are on vacation? Last year, I actually lost weight while we were on a Mediterranean cruise for ten days. Great food selections were always available and many opportunities for exercise (shipboard and shore side). Sure, you can cheat here and there (now that you know the technique) but the main thing is to enjoy yourself, relax and look for opportunities to strengthen your new habits.

- *"I'm not an athlete so I can't work out or go to the gym..."*
You can get a great workout, even if you're totally non-athletic. Get started with simple walking. Plus, there are many great exercises you can do in the comfort of your own home, just using

your own body weight… no equipment necessary (see Chapter 13).

- *"My friends eat junk food so it's hard for me…"*
  I agree that, it is difficult when you are constantly around people who are eating poorly. It can certainly be done, but if it is too hard for you, it may mean spending less time with these people. Some of my clients have found that taking this somewhat drastic measure was the only path to success. Think this one through carefully and make the best decision, considering you and your health as <u>priority number one</u>.

- *"I hate to exercise because it makes me hungry…"*
  I love this one! I heard a famous radio broadcaster use this one the other day too. The whole point of exercise is to build lean muscle tissue and consume more energy than you are taking in with food. If you are feeling real hunger pangs, that's good. It means you didn't overeat at your last meal and it means you are losing weight. Celebrate and eat a healthy snack – you deserve it!

- *"I blew it today, so I'll get started again next Monday..."*
  This used to be a pretty good excuse for you, eh? Not anymore. You will learn and memorize the **No Fear™** cheating technique (Chapter Six) which means you will get back on your healthy eating program *immediately*.

- *"I'll just sleep for a few minutes longer..."*
  This is one of my favorites because I use it more frequently than I should (particularly in the winter months). Fortunately for me, I have the schedule flexibility to get my butt out of bed a little later and then get out the door. If you can juggle your schedule, great. If not, get up and get moving... sooner than you think, you'll be looking forward to your workouts.

Nowhere to Run, Nowhere to Hide
Well, you've just run the gauntlet of excuses and here you are, out in the sunshine. Nowhere to run, nowhere to hide and most importantly, you have **no excuses**!

A critical concept in the *Weight Loss for Wimps™ System* is that of *taking personal responsibility* for your current situation and your future. And that means removing all the obstacles in your path. A lame, wimpy excuse is one of those obstacles that must be squashed like a bug.

It's fine to acknowledge your past mistakes and even acknowledge what others may have done to you. However, to move forward towards your **Big Dream**, you must stay focused on your future - the future that *you* will create for yourself.

Do we have a deal? Let's shake hands on it to seal the deal, ok?

**Weight Loss for Wimps™
Success Step Seven**

> <u>**Attitude**</u>: I refuse to give up on my **Big Dream**.
>
> I will do whatever it takes to change my lifestyle habits to get healthy and reach my perfect weight.
>
> <u>**Skills**</u>: I have carefully reviewed the list of common, wimpy excuses and although I see one or more that I use to justify my current

weight situation, I agree that none of them apply to me.

I have entered the "No Excuses Zone"

Action: Make note in your daily journal the top three excuses you have used to justify not starting or staying on a healthy lifestyle program.

Look yourself in the mirror and repeat out loud,
"I have No Excuses!"

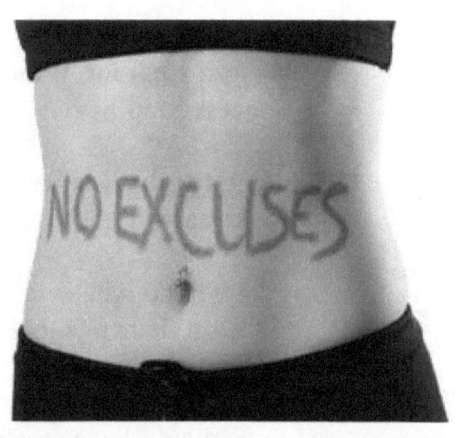

CHAPTER EIGHT

TACTICS FOR DEALING WITH EMOTIONAL EATING

EMOTIONAL EATING AND his cousin, Stress are the "all-stars" on the opposing team, determined to defeat your efforts to win the game and get healthy, sexy and thin. We'll study their moves carefully and lay out a specific game plan to annihilate them - take them both totally out of the game for good.

In this chapter we'll focus on emotional eating exclusively and then discuss stress in the following chapter.

Before we get into the details, I want to put this somewhat delicate topic of emotional eating into context. I use the term "delicate" because some people become very defensive, dismissive and even angry when this subject is raised. I found this out almost immediately when I started working with my private coaching clients.

And by the way, if you're a Manly Man and think that only women have emotional eating issues… you are dead wrong. These issues are just as common with men; it's just that you may

125

be more skilled at hiding them. So pay attention!

Emotional eating is not a psychiatric condition requiring medical treatment, nor is it a secret social stigma that you should keep hidden to avoid ridicule (Note that some specific eating disorders such as bulimia or anorexia *are* conditions that require professional medical expertise and you should seek immediate treatment if you suffer from one of these conditions).

On the contrary, emotional eating is a common, internal adversary that almost all of us overweight folks have to learn to deal with and defeat. Many academics and weight loss coaching practitioners feel this is the <u>number one</u> cause of obesity and diet failure.

One of the preeminent medical authorities on this subject, Roger Gould, M.D. from UCLA studied over 17,000 failed dieters and concluded that virtually *all* of them ultimately relapsed *because they lacked the skills needed to deal with emotional eating.*

Don't worry; I'm going to teach you the skills you need to crush this adversary…

But first, let's find out a little more about this bad boy called **emotional eating**.

Emotional Eating Basics
What is emotional eating?

In a nutshell, emotional eating is characterized by habitually and suddenly eating when you are not physically hungry and is triggered by your mind's response to an emotion that you would rather not feel.

In other words, it is the use of food to soothe or comfort feelings, rather than experiencing the emotion and then dealing with the triggering person, place or event.

Another key characteristic of emotional eating is that shortly after you wolf down that chocolate candy bar, bag of potato chips or pint of ice cream (or all three)… you _always_ feel like a total, wimpy loser. You hate yourself for not having the willpower or self-discipline to control your eating. You're disgusted with yourself. It felt so incredibly good for a little while going down, but afterwards, not so much.

This is much, much different than using the _No Fear_™ cheating technique discussed in Chapter Six. That was all about planning a cheating episode in advance, which is your goal if you're going to stray from your plan.

In contrast, emotional eating is about dealing with an almost uncontrollable, sudden urge to sprint to the vending machine to grab a Snicker's bar (or whatever your favorite comfort food is), because you didn't get invited to go to lunch with some of your co-workers today; or maybe you just found out that you didn't make it on the short list for this Friday night's poker game?

Dealing with hurt feelings vs. a Snicker's bar... no brainer, the Snicker's bar, right?

The problem is, until you've been trained, it is typically not a decision making process. You just go eat, and then think about it later, with much regret. This is the part that we will focus our attention on - breaking up this "auto-pilot" response.

Uncomfortable Emotions and Uncomfortable Triggers
We don't like to feel angry, hurt, upset, unloved, disappointed, envious, lonely, grief, frustration, fear... these are not "happy" thoughts and we would prefer to spend as much time in the "happy mode" as possible.

On the other hand, these so called negative emotions are <u>normal</u> human signals that we need to listen to and learn to respond to with appropriate behaviors. As mature adults, we need to recognize that these emotions are the doorway into our "inner self", which is where all the action is.

Once we allow ourselves to enter into the arena of our "inner self" we can quietly, carefully, methodically think through logical options and plan out an appropriate behavioral response. This is where alternatives are evaluated, problems are solved and action plans are developed. Personally, I think of it as the "war room", but that's probably a guy thing; use an analogy you like - maybe the "castle" or the "sanctuary" or the "retreat". Think of it as a place of peace, quiet reflection and safety.

If you consistently shut-down this doorway by using food to "escape", you never get inside the arena to consider options. You bypass the problem-solving step altogether, but the problem doesn't go away. It just lurks in the shadows, awaiting the opportunity to resurface. That's the insidious nature of this emotional eating bad boy - one of his trick plays that he will use at every opportunity.

One of the primary trick plays in his "bag of tricks" is to use situations, places or events to trigger one of the uncomfortable emotions so he can get you headed to the buffet table instead of the goal line… the classic head fake misdirection play.

For example, maybe every time you go on a "girl's night out" ritual, you totally blow it, without restriction. You pound down the margaritas, inhale the pasta and bread and can't wait to order the "death by chocolate" dessert.

There are an endless number of other possible situations, places or events that for you, could trigger one or more of the uncomfortable emotions; weddings, funerals, social events, job interviews, job performance reviews, class reunions, weekly staff meetings, company parties, etc. Think and start making your list.

But this emotional eating dude inside your head is no ordinary player. He's an "all star" for a reason… and he reserves his best trick play by using other people in your life. It could be your wife, ex-husband, boss, boyfriend, girlfriend, kids, "friend", neighbor, co-worker, mother, mother-in-law, or sister; in fact, any of the people with whom you interact with on a regular basis.

Something is said…or not said… something is done or not done… or it could be a look or a glance in your direction… it could be a late arrival or no arrival at all. Whatever it is, this person gets under your skin and sets off your uncomfortable emotions like a firecracker on New Year's Eve.

Your mother-in-law shows up at your house for a two day visit and you immediately start slurping down Coke's (with maybe a little rum added). You can't seem to do anything right in her eyes. She's constantly making snide little remarks… and you're biting your tongue to keep the peace.

What other choice do you have but to self medicate with your own favorite selection of over-the-counter food drugs?

It gets you through the situation. You'll survive for another day. As soon as the grumpy old woman (GOW) leaves, things will return to normal (although you may have gained another 5 lbs).

When you're under the influence of this emotional eating power player, it doesn't even occur to you that you have other options. The emotion-food relationship is hard wired and on auto pilot. The emotion pops up and you pop up, and head straight for the refrigerator.

We're going to change that emotion-food relationship and we're going after that hard wiring connection with a sledge hammer and a vengeance. This "all star" is about to get whacked and sent down to the minor leagues!

The *I Learn*™ To End Emotional Eating Technique
Follow me closely on this one and you will forever change your relationship with food and will learn to calmly crush emotional eating every time he raises his ugly head in the future.

It will require some intense practice over time but just like any skill, your proficiency will grow by leaps and bounds with a little persistence.

In developing my *I Learn*™ technique, I have relied heavily on the self discovery process during my own weight loss journey. Recall that after weight loss camp, I was on my own to figure out how to stay on track. Unfortunately, I didn't receive any skills training on this issue at camp.

But I had emotional eating issues, just like everybody else. As I tried different ideas, things eventually started falling into place. Later on, I began working with my coaching clients and I began to further research the topic in the popular press and in various scientific resources. The *I Learn™* technique that follows is my synthesis of this effort:

Let's briefly describe each step so you can implement and practice these skills in order to nail this emotional eating dude to the wall:

1. Identify Your Emotional Eating Behaviors

Yes, it is *theoretically* possible that you do not have any emotional eating issues. Let's find out, one way or the other.

I want you to think back about your meals and snacks over the past day or two and answer these questions:

- At any time, did you actually feel hungry prior to eating or was it just 6 pm and time to eat?

- Do you normally feel hunger in your stomach or is it more often located in your mouth or throat?

- Did the feeling of hunger occur suddenly with great intensity?

- Did you eat when you were upset, angry, frustrated or disappointed?

- Did you finish your meals in seven minutes or less?

- Did you eat all of the food that was served i.e. did you clean your plate?

- Did you go back for a second helping of any food item? Or, did you finish food leftover on your spouse or kids' plates?

- Did you have any feelings of guilt or regret after you ate?

- Did you have any cravings for a particular food or treat?

As a recovering emotional eater myself, I know the tendency to rationalize. Be brutally honest with yourself in answering those questions.

I'm going to abbreviate the term "emotional eater's" with "EE's" in commenting on these questions:

At any time, did you actually feel hungry prior to eating or was it just 6 pm and time to eat?
EE's typically do not wait until they feel real physical hunger; that feeling is to be avoided at all costs! And we normally eat by the clock.

Do you normally feel hunger in your stomach or is it more often located in your mouth or throat?
For many EE's, physical hunger is a foreign concept (it sure was for me personally). Instead, EE's will experience "fake" or "phantom" hunger that is usually felt in your mouth or throat, not your belly.

Did the feeling of hunger occur suddenly with great intensity?
One of the key characteristics of EE is a sudden and an almost uncontrollable urge to eat following an emotional event. EE's often feel there is no other choice but to eat.

Did you eat when you were upset, angry, frustrated or disappointed?

This is the hallmark characteristic of EE's.

Did you finish your meals in 7 minutes or less?

EE's eat very quickly, almost "inhaling" the food. The fork or spoon never leaves the hand!

Did you eat all of the food that was served i.e. did you clean your plate?

Most of us that overeat will eat all of the food that is served (unless there is a particular item that we dislike). This is an issue at home when serving ourselves, because we tend to match the "super-sized" portions we receive at most restaurants. We consider these giant portions to be normal or otherwise acceptable.

Did you go back for a second helping of any food item? Or, did you finish food leftover on your spouses or kids' plates?

This was always one of my personal favorite overeating techniques. Of course we're not physically hungry; in fact we're probably stuffed after finishing our own oversized meal... but we can't let the rest of that hamburger go to waste! Gobble, gobble.

Did you have any feelings of guilt or regret after you ate?

EE's always feel guilty after an eating frenzy or binge. We always regret what we ate and how much we ate.

Did you have any cravings for a particular food or treat?

EE's usually get intense cravings for a particular comfort food...a healthy snack or healthy meal is just not on the list of something that will satisfy the craving.

How did you do on the quiz? Do you feel that your emotions *may* play *some* role in your eating patterns? If not, you can move on to the next chapter - otherwise, continue with the next step.

2. Listen to Your Emotional Signals and Triggers

This step is crucial in gaining an understanding of your mind-body connection. You need to know the source of your negative feelings. Over the next few weeks, whenever you get that irresistible urge for your comfort food, jot down in your journal the 'who, what, when, where' so you can shine the light on these trouble spots. These are the triggers – people, places, situations, events – that stimulate your overwhelming desire for food, regardless of your true state of hunger.

Be sure to include *yourself* as a possible trigger. EE's are often self-critical and can create the burning desire for food without the need for external stimulus. It's important to make note of this situation too.

Remember, in this step you are beginning to learn to become self-aware of how your thoughts, feelings, and body interact under a variety of circumstances. Work on this list every day until you think you have most of your common situations noted in your journal. The idea here is to build an inventory so that you can think through and be prepared to deal with these circumstances in the future.

3. Experience the Emotion – Go to Your Inner Sanctuary
This is the centerpiece of the *I Learn*™ process.

You must learn to accept negative emotions as "normal" and let them flow to the surface and experience them. <u>Do not suppress them</u>. <u>Do not fear them.</u>

Are you angry? Let it out and express it in a situational/socially appropriate way (no finger signals out on the highway!).

Do you feel like crying? Cry! Cry for as long as it takes to get it out. You'll feel ten times better once you do it.

Particularly in a work setting, my clients and I have found that going to the bathroom and getting in a stall is an almost ideal location to let your emotions flow. Regardless, find an environment of peace and quiet and relative isolation. Now, you have the privacy you need and...

You have created the most important aspect of this process – a break in time – an interruption of the hard wiring that currently exists in your emotion-food circuit.

When you're ready, take a deep breath, compose yourself and allow yourself to enter the arena of your *inner self*. This is your inner "sanctuary", or in my case the "war room", where you can quietly begin to reflect on the situation that triggered the emotion.

139

4. <u>A</u>nalyze Your Options and Take Action
As you carefully, calmly and quietly begin to evaluate options for handling the situation, there are a couple of key questions you can ask yourself in almost any scenario:

a. Is this a situation over which I have no control?

For example, a friend or loved one passed away. You obviously have no control over this situation. Nevertheless, it stimulates various emotions that you need to work through, *without resorting to eating.* Life presents us with many challenges wherein we really have no control. The stock market crashes, the company we work for goes bankrupt, our parents develop serious medical conditions, our house is destroyed in a hurricane, etc. In other words, this type of situation requires ***coping skills***, not **problem solving skills**. My best advice in a coping situation is to seek help and advice from family and friends. Reach out and talk to others…they are anxious to help you get through the situation.

b. Is this a situation over which you do have partial or full control?

For example, you are in a job that you absolutely hate. Your boss is a jerk   and your job duties are boring beyond human endurance. You're constantly anxious, frustrated, short-tempered, and can't stand your boss's secretary.

This situation requires ***problem solving skills***. It's something you do have   control over. You have options. You have the ability to make reasoned choices. You can quit, transfer, look for a new job, start your own business, seek a promotion, seek new and exciting job duties… the list goes on.

In most problem solving situations, ask yourself these questions:

Is there another way to view this situation that I may not have considered? What is it? If I changed my view, how would that impact the problem? Did my behavior contribute to this problem?

All sides considered, what is the most likely outcome of this situation?

What would I tell my best friend or a close family member to do in this same situation?

What should I do *right now* to move forward and get this resolved?

This is your action item. Make that phone call, schedule that appointment, ask for a meeting, set up a lunch date, call the school, call a time-out… and then take another deep breath and put a smile on your face.

You've made a positive step in the right direction and did so *without food*… so give yourself a well deserved pat on the back!

You're probably still a little upset or down in the dumps, but at least you did something positive that will likely lead to a final resolution.

Do you have some time *right now* to take a little break?

5. <u>R</u>elief Valve

It's important that as soon as possible after you've thought through your situation and made the first step to address the issue, that you take a little break. Get your mind focused on something enjoyable, even for five minutes, just to relieve some of the pressure.

The list of potential activities is almost endless. Experiment with a variety of relaxation and distraction activities that you find enjoyable…maybe you'll even find one that involves a bit of exercise (hint, hint!):

Take the dog for a walk	E-mail a joke to a friend	Go window shopping
Ride your bike	Take a yoga or Pilates class	Listen to some music
Go for a jog	Do a Sudoku puzzle	Work on a crafts project
Give your dog a bath	Play Guitar Hero	Practice your instrument
Go to the gym	Work on your scrapbook	Elevator down; walk up
Take a tennis lesson	Play 9 holes of golf	Hit a bucket at the range

Mix and match and try new activities. Find out which activities work best for you. The idea is to relieve some pressure and to keep your mind occupied…*and not thinking about food!*

6. <u>N</u>urture a New Relationship With Food

As a serial overeater and emotional eater, I had to eventually come to grips with the concept that "I do <u>not</u> have a healthy, wholesome relationship with food."

I used food as a delivery mechanism to "get a temporary high" to "feel good", much like a drug or alcohol addict. I had my favorite drugs (chips, burgers, french fries, bread, Coke and Oreo or chocolate chip cookies served with whole milk). But at times, just about any junk food within reach was good enough…it got the job done.

Fruits and vegetables? Forget it…they were just bothersome little side dishes that got in the way of the main course.

No wonder I ultimately ballooned up to almost 300 lbs; could hardly walk, popping nitroglycerin pills… and thinking about death and dying every day. Not a pretty picture. You've read my story earlier and know the struggles I went through.

I cannot emphasize enough the importance of developing a healthy relationship with *good* food. You simply cannot get to where you need and want to be… healthy, sexy and thin…

without establishing a new attitude and belief system about good, healthy food. This has to be done at the conscious and subconscious mind levels.

At the same time, you will have to make the transition to developing a strong negative attitude and rejection towards unhealthy junk food, including high sugar sodas and other drinks.

Does that scare you? Does that mean you can never, ever enjoy any of the foods you love now? Of course not. Total deprivation of any particular food is a sure recipe for weight loss failure.

You've already learned how to cheat successfully using the *No Fear*™ protocol discussed in Chapter 6. The idea though, is to use that technique very sparingly because eventually you want to wean yourself off all the crap food entirely...or almost entirely.

> *"That sounds good on paper, but exactly how do I suddenly change my attitudes and beliefs about food?"*

It didn't happen for me *suddenly* and I don't expect it will for you either. Like anything worthwhile, it takes a little time and effort. Cultivate your new relationship day by day. As we discussed earlier, bad habits and thought patterns are difficult to break. Nobody said it would be easy.

But what I've done to help you is to develop a simple, short set of beliefs and attitudes about food that I want you to consider adopting as your own. Review them, repeat them, and eventually make them become a part of you.

Belief and attitude are a hundred times stronger than willpower.

I call my belief system the *I Love™ Good Food Philosophy:*

The *I Love™ Good Food* Philosophy

I eat *good* food because what I eat determines the health and strength of every cell in my body.

Lifestyle – *good* food provides the fuel I need to burn excess fat and to create an energetic, active lifestyle.

146

Obesity and illness are defeated by eliminating highly processed "fake" foods that are damaging my health and preventing me from reaching my perfect weight.

Very little effort is required to select *good*, high quality food that I can use to prepare delicious and satisfying gourmet meals.

Every nutrient I need for perfect health is available in *good* food.

Instinctively, you already know the difference between *good* food and junk food or unhealthy food. Nevertheless, we'll dive into that subject more fully in the Chapters found in Part Three.

Let me ask you to do me a favor, ok?

I'd like you to sit back, close your eyes for a few minutes, and just think about your prior battles with emotional eating. Can you see how powerful this guy has been in your life?

Now, I'd like you to think about the new skills you've learned in this Chapter. You have in your hands and mind all the counter-moves and offensive plays needed to whip this guy and send him packing to the minor leagues.

You have the power and the skills to win every battle. Use it or lose it. Now!

Weight Loss for Wimps™
Success Step Eight

> **Attitude**: I acknowledge that emotional eating is a powerful force in my life that must be defeated.
>
> I have consistently struggled with how to effectively deal with my emotions but I am determined to do so without using food.
>
> I have <u>not</u> had a healthy, wholesome relationship with food but am committed to forever changing that relationship.
>
> **Skills**: I will implement each of the six steps in the *I Learn™ to End Emotional Eating* process.
>
> I will incorporate into my daily life the *I Love™ Good Food Philosophy* to permanently change my relationship with food.
>
> **Action**: Carefully study the details of the *I Learn™* process; document the six steps in

your daily journal. Begin recording the emotional triggers you encounter over the next few weeks. Make special notes about your successes in implementing these new skills.

Review the *I Love™ Good Food* Philosophy on a daily basis. Record these beliefs and attitudes in your journal. Consider posting them on your refrigerator door.

CHAPTER NINE

TACTICS FOR DEALING WITH STRESS

STRESS IS THE "ALL STAR" teammate of emotional eating. They work hand-in-hand together to block your efforts to reach the goal line and achieve the healthy, sexy, thin body and your **Big Dream**.

Like emotional eating, stress wants you to eat when you are not hungry and urges you to gobble down readily available comfort food to soothe your frazzled nerves.

But stress has his very own special trick play that we will focus on in this Chapter; I call it his "deer in the headlights" play. We'll get into how to defend against that play in a few minutes.

First, let's learn more about this opponent so we can gain a better understanding of how he operates in real life.

Stress 101
Stress is not "what happens to us." Rather, stress is about *"how we respond to what happens to us in our day-to-day living."*

Similar to emotional eating, it's a reflection of our individual ability to *cope* with difficult situations or events outside of our control (job loss, illness, death in the family) and our ability to *solve the daily problems* within our control (arriving to work on time, getting the car serviced, cleaning the kitchen, balancing our checkbook, dealing with a failed relationship or problem child).

One of the key distinguishing features of stress is that it results in immediate biochemical changes in our body. Adrenalin and related hormones are quickly released which increases our heart rate, blood pressure, blood sugar, inflammation and our blood clotting. These are normal, healthy bodily responses designed into our fight-or-flight physiology that saves our lives by allowing us to respond effectively when dealing with crowding, danger, infection, or extremes of temperature.

Problems related to stress occur when we are chronically and repeatedly subjected to stress over time. Medical research has clearly shown that chronic, unresolved stress can result in a variety of debilitating physical illnesses such as heart disease, insulin resistance leading to diabetes, high blood pressure, osteoporosis and perhaps even cancer. Unresolved stress is obviously serious and deadly, apart from its contribution to our eating issues.

Stress is a fact of life… living is periodically stressful… and all of us <u>must</u> learn the skills to deal with it effectively. That means improving our stress related coping skills and problem solving skills (more on this later).

The Stress–Eating Connection
For our purposes, we will focus on how stress, if not handled properly, can quickly lead us down the path to stuffing ourselves with large volumes of very unhealthy food - pizza, chocolate candy, monster burgers, soda, alcohol, and other comfort foods of choice.

The complication with chronic stress-induced eating is that is does have a physiological basis. With prolonged stress, an additional hormone called *cortisol* is released in high amounts, which like adrenaline, also increases blood pressure and blood sugar. *And it can result in a significant increase in appetite*. Unfortunately, the cellular receptors for cortisol are located in our abdomen, which triggers fat storage leading to increased risk of metabolic syndrome and other illnesses discussed previously.

This stress-eating response applies to both sexes but women are particularly vulnerable, according to recent research at the University of California at San Francisco. In their studies, the researchers found that women who eat higher-fat diets were shown to have both an increase in cortisol reaction and a greater preference for sweet foods in response to stress. Ouch!

There is also evidence to suggest that excess cortisol can slow down our metabolism in an effort to conserve energy. This then, can result in an eat more-burn less "double-whammy" when under the influence of prolonged periods of stress. Double ouch!

Conclusion: stress cannot only kill you, before it does that, it can make you fat! Let's figure out how to better handle stressful situations in our daily lives.

Stress Coping Skills
Recall that coping skills are applicable to stress induced situations that are generated by events beyond our control. They just happen and we need to work through the situation, instead of going for the brownie and ice cream (one of my favorites!).

Common situations would include a relationship breakup, death or sudden severe illness in the family or of a close friend, sudden behavioral issues with your kids, increased workload or new deadlines at your job. Usually, these can be viewed as temporary situations that with a little time and most importantly outside *support*, will resolve themselves.

The key skill to use in these situations is to actively seek out support from family and or friends. Reach out and find people who are willing to spend time with you to just talk. Without a doubt, this is the most powerful remedy for calming your nerves and working through the disappointment, fear and or hurt.

The absolute worst thing you can do is turn inward and socially isolate yourself from people in your sphere. This leads inevitably to bitterness, anger, hate, mistrust, and of course, food.

Seek out people who see the glass as half full, who are fun to be around, who like to laugh. These are emotionally nourishing people who offer unconditional affection, friendship, love, humor and perpetual optimism. Hang with these people because they will help you get through your crisis and steer you in the direction of understanding, fulfillment and happiness.

Deflate Your Self-Inflicted Lifestyle Stress
In the previous chapter on emotional eating, we discussed problem solving skills for situations that you have partial or full control over. With a little practice, you can use those skills to make significant progress on just about any stressful situation you encounter. Review the *I Learn™* techniques again, with particular attention to the problem solving skills in step four, *Analyze Your Options and Take Action*.

However, the issue I want to discuss here is what I call self-induced or self-inflicted lifestyle stress. This is stress we bring on ourselves due to our day-to-day choices.

Let's face it…many of us, particularly those of us in North America are stress junkies. We purposely live life on the edge of emotional and financial disaster. We work 80 hours a week at a job we despise yet we lust for the corner office with windows (out of the cubicles); we crave and buy the largest house in the fanciest neighborhood possible; we play office and social politics to maximize our exposure; we carpool and taxi our kids to six different after school activities; we volunteer to coach the kids' soccer team and help with the room mother duties at school; then, because our finances are maxed out, we dabble in dubious schemes with dreams of building a six-figure "part-time" income that is a total waste of our little remaining precious time and financial resources.

In between all this, we have to deal with trying to maintain our daily responsibilities of actual living - grocery shopping, dentist appointments, teacher-parent meetings, mowing the lawn, washing the dishes, paying the bills, getting the tires rotated on the car… blah, blah, yada, yada…

And the result of all this is incredible, sustained, unrelenting, chronic <u>stress</u>. No wonder our cortisol levels are off the chart and we crave junk food like a starving refugee.

Inevitably, we get to the point of being positively, absolutely, <u>overwhelmed</u> resulting in what I call "*the deer in the headlights syndrome.*" This is the special trick play that our opponent, Stress has up his sleeve. And it can be a game changer.

When you're driving along the country road at night (in an area that has deer), you occasionally come upon a deer in the middle of the road. The deer turns its head toward you and all of a sudden just *freezes* in place; the headlights are blinding, the animal is confused, and doesn't know what to do; the uncertainty and stress causes its mind and body to just shut-down, frozen in time.

The same thing can happen to us humans, if we *allow* ourselves to become so stressed out and overwhelmed that we just shut-down our cognitive thinking ability; we can't make reasoned decisions, we can't keep commitments, we misplace important items or papers, we can't sleep, we are confused as to which direction to go, and our emotions control our lives. When our enemies, Emotional Eating and Stress, work in tandem to gain the upper hand; we eat, and eat, and eat whatever we can quickly get our hands on. The *last thing* we have on our minds is healthy, mindful eating and exercise - game over.

The solution is so simple, so obvious that it <u>*screams*</u> for implementation:

Simplify Your Life!

The most important skill that you can develop and implement right now, this very moment, is to *learn and practice the skill of saying "No!"*

This is very difficult for some people, particularly nurturing, caring personalities who thrive on pleasing other people. But it is a critical skill to develop because your health and sanity (and weight loss goals) depend on it.

Learn to prioritize your day-to-day activities. Actively look for anything and everything that you can eliminate from your life that is unnecessarily eating up your precious time and in some cases, your financial resources. Get rid of them permanently or at least defer them to some future date when you may have more time available.

Deflate the stress in your life by simplification. What is mission critical and what is not. Focus on the most important aspects of your life and get rid of the rest because they are impacting your ability to create a healthy lifestyle.

It gets back to the message in Chapter Four – *Making You Priority One*.

Getting rid of the clutter in your daily life will not only remove much of the chronic stress you have allowed in, it will free up significant blocks of time that can be used for any of the relaxation and distraction activities discussed in the previous chapter.

And it provides you the necessary time to carefully plan and cook healthy meals for you and your family and time to exercise your body. Exercise, by the way, is perhaps the best stress reliever available. If nothing else, take a walk!

A few more quick tips to consider:

- Review and make notes in your daily journal every evening prior to going to bed. This will help you relax, reflect on accomplishments, make note of problem areas and get you focused on tomorrow.

- Try to get at least seven hours of sleep each night. New research shows the benefits of this habit on weight loss efforts.

- Plan your day the night before.

- Go to bed at least 15 minutes earlier and get up at least 15 minutes earlier. This allows you a little more time to get yourself organized for the day and to make sure you have a relaxed, healthy breakfast.

I hope that you are feeling more empowered to effectively deal with the dynamic duo of emotional eating and stress. Yes, they are powerful and tricky. But you now have the framework and ability to develop the skills to knock them out of the game. Take action and implement.

In the next chapter, we'll work on the all important issue of hunger, both real and imagined, and how to effectively handle this, our final adversary.

**Weight Loss for Wimps™
Success Step Nine**

> **<u>Attitude</u>**: I acknowledge that I sometimes don't handle unexpected stressful situations very well and use food to help calm my nerves.
>
> I also acknowledge that I have over-committed some of my time to unnecessary activities that I can live without.
>
> I feel at times that I am overwhelmed.

<u>Skills</u>: When I face an unexpected crisis, I will seek out loving and supporting people who can help me. I will not try to do it alone.

I am committed to simplifying my lifestyle in order to focus on the important tasks. I will eliminate superfluous activities to create blocks of time to relax, relieve stress and to develop healthy eating and exercise habits.

I will say "<u>No</u>" often, with a smile on my face and without guilt.

<u>Action</u>: Make a list in your journal of specific activities that you will eliminate immediately. Be ruthless! Also list those tasks that you can delegate to others or that you can phase out quickly.

Starting today, record in your journal when you said "<u>No</u>".

Make new friends with funny, happy people!

CHAPTER TEN

TACTICS FOR DEALING WITH HUNGER

HUNGER IS THE ULTIMATE enemy you will face in your day to day battles to reach your **Big Dream** and obtain the healthy, sexy, and thin body you always wanted and deserve.

This bad boy is like no other that we've discussed previously. He is so tricky, so nefarious that we place him in a special category - *Most Valuable Player* on the Super Bowl or World Cup team that we are playing against. He is that good.

While emotional eating is certainly powerful and has been labeled as the most important cause of obesity, hunger is often given the special place of honor in the Hall of Fame as *the most important cause of diet failure.*

The Special Powers of Hunger
What is it about hunger that makes this opponent so important and powerful?

Hunger comes at us on two distinct levels: (1) *real physical hunger,* when your stomach "growls" or your body otherwise signals a physiological need for food; and (2) *fake hunger*, oftentimes felt as a sensation in your mouth or throat area (like when you salivate thinking about a Big Mac) but is not a true physiological hunger signal. It's just the trickster trying to get you to eat when you are not hungry and when you don't need the additional calorie input.

In order for us to win our daily battles with hunger, we must first be able to recognize and distinguish the two forms. Easy to do, now that you know the difference, right?

Just knowing that these two forms of hunger exist is a huge advantage for you – most people don't have a clue and are unable to make the distinction; they mistakenly assume that hunger is hunger. We'll discuss specific tactics momentarily.

First, let's discuss the unique power hunger can exert over us.

The power that hunger has over us as individuals' stems mostly from our cultural *fear of hunger* and learned behavior to *avoid hunger*, at all costs.

In most Western cultures, hunger is a sign of poverty and therefore something to be avoided. This is a gross over-simplification but gets to the point. We abhor the feeling of hunger because it is uncomfortable physically, socially and psychologically because it is associated with inner-city poverty or third world living conditions.

I don't want to go off the deep end into psycho-babble, but, in essence, we are conditioned from early childhood to avoid physical hunger and we generally associate food and fullness with a loving, caring, parental environment.

There is nothing inherently wrong with this attitude because we want our children to love good food and develop into strong, healthy young adults.

Diet Industry Malpractice
The problem comes in when we are trying to break the overeating cycle and trying to lose the excess weight we've accumulated. What I am about to share with you may be quite *shocking* because it is contrary to what everyone in the weight loss industry always tells you…

The idea of losing weight
and never feeling hungry

are in fact, mutually exclusive concepts. It is almost impossible to lose weight and never feel hungry

This "minor little detail" is always brushed aside by the diet industry because they know that they can't get you in the door unless they promise,

"You'll never feel hungry on our diet!"

This is a real disservice, bordering on malpractice. Instead of teaching you about hunger and how to deal with it effectively, they ignore the issue altogether or make it sound like something is wrong with *you* if you get hungry on their diet.

The cold, hard reality is this: When losing weight *and* when you are in maintenance mode, you will experience brief periods of real physical hunger, probably on a daily basis.

How I Discovered Hunger Is My Friend
As you recall my story, I was having trouble losing weight and staying on a sensible eating plan. That's when I casually thought out loud, "Maybe I should go to a fat camp..." My wife

overheard my musings and the next thing I know, I'm on a plane going to a weight loss camp in South Carolina for three weeks.

I was *immediately* placed on a 1,200 calorie per day diet and I was *immediately* hungry…

Upon reflection, since I had a lot of free time on my hands over three weeks, I couldn't remember the last time I actually experienced real hunger. Maybe it was during our Peace Corps days in Cameroon, Africa, far removed from our normal Western diet; or maybe during my military training…

In any event, it was a very long time ago because I, like most overweight people, never allowed myself to even come close to being "stomach growling" hungry. I overate at every meal and in between meals too, just to make sure I never experienced hunger.

Every day at camp, for three weeks, I experienced stomach growling hunger, at least a couple of times a day. This was something new and I thought for sure, my stomach was going to shrink so that I eventually wouldn't feel hungry. That didn't happen.

Once I returned home from camp to real life, I had a problem. How to deal with the hunger I was facing every day.

It's one thing to be in a closed environment like weight loss camp (or military boot camp) where choices are made for you. It's another thing to be back home in an open environment where you have to make choices for yourself.

I instinctively knew that I had to develop a new mindset on the issue of feeling hungry. Here's what I came up with that has worked very well for me and my coaching clients; I call it my *Hunger Is Good™ Mindset.*

When I feel stomach growling hunger and I know it's <u>not</u> an appropriate meal or snack time, I talk to myself as follows:

- "It's good that I feel hungry… it means that I didn't overeat at the last meal"

- "It's good that I feel hungry… it means that I am taking in less calories than I'm burning, which means I'm losing weight"

- "I'll just ignore the hunger pangs because they will go away in just a few minutes anyway. I can wait until my normal meal time... it's no big deal"

Adopting the *Hunger Is Good™ Mindset* was crucial to my success in weight loss and is an important theme in the *Weight Loss for Wimps™ System*. Another way to look at hunger in this context is as follows:

> **If we *fear hunger* and do everything and anything to *avoid hunger*, we lose - we lose the game, not the weight!**

Tactics For Dealing With Real Hunger

Incorporate the *Hunger Is Good™ Mindset* into your daily thought processes. Learn to accept that physical hunger is a signal from your body that you are doing things correctly, getting healthy and losing weight.

You will quickly discover, as did I, that the hunger pangs typically do not last very long. In addition, there are a number of activities you can use to distract yourself from thinking about your hunger:

168

- Drink plenty of water
- Go for a quick walk

- Call a friend
- Think about your **Big Dream**

Since the day I arrived at weight loss camp through and including today (almost four years and 88 lbs later), I feel physical hunger every day. I have learned to expect it and now recognize it as "normal."

Over the past few months, I've been casually conducting an informal survey of **thin** people I encounter.

"During the course of a normal day, do you ever feel real hunger pangs, like stomach growling hunger pangs?"

The overwhelming response can be summarized as follows...

"Yes, of course, doesn't everybody? Sometimes I just forget to eat, so I'll grab a piece of fruit or hand full of nuts; something to hold me over until my next meal."

This is how a naturally thin, mindful eater thinks. Feeling hungry is not the end of the world!

Fighting Real Hunger With Real Food
Real hunger is also effectively managed by including certain foods in your diet that provide a sense of fullness (satiety) and that are more slowly metabolized into your bloodstream.

These include foods that are high in fiber such as cereals, oatmeal, high-fiber breads, beans, blackberries or raspberries, walnuts and green vegetables like broccoli. Fiber is especially valuable in a healthy diet because it stabilizes your blood chemistry and significantly helps your weight loss efforts by extending your feeling of fullness. Look for opportunities to add fiber at each meal, up to about 40 grams per day.

Research has demonstrated that including a high-protein meal component significantly slows down the return to the hunger state. In other words, protein is metabolized at a much slower rate than carbohydrates so you stay satisfied for a much longer period of time. Fish has been found to be particularly effective in this role.

Another favorite technique is to include a large volume salad with a low calorie dressing and a bowl of soup with high density grains (barley) or vegetables. These are excellent menu choices for both managing your hunger and managing your calories.

Tactics For Dealing With Fake Hunger
Fake hunger or as some researchers call it, *phantom hunger,* is simply your mind responding to some external factor like an emotional situation or a stress event by getting you to eat when you're not really hungry. As we've discussed earlier, you can distinguish this urge to eat by noting that the sensation can be traced to your mouth or throat area rather than your stomach. It feels more like "mouth watering" or salivating when thinking about food.

The tactics for dealing with fake hunger are identical to the *I Learn*™ process for emotional eating and the *I Love*™ *Good Food* thought process for establishing a new, healthy relationship with good food.

The key is to recognize the fake hunger play when it happens and then stop it cold in its tracks. Diversion, distraction, movement, activity - just keep going, ignoring fake hunger because without attention, he will disappear very quickly.

Lately, one of my favorite counter-moves is to pop a stick of sugarless gum into my mouth. It seems to satisfy any cravings, take my mind off food and allow me to get focused on something else. Give it try… it may work for you, too.

Circling The Wagons

You've now been introduced to the "Four Bad Boys" that are out to ruin your efforts to get healthy, sexy and thin - excuses, emotional eating, stress and hunger. They will be on the field every day, testing you, prodding you, jerking you around.

But, you've got their number. You know their moves, you know when they are likely to appear and best of all, you know how to defeat them each and every time. You have learned the skills that when practiced, honed and implemented consistently, will catapult you to enter the winner's circle.

The **Big Dream** is not only possible, it is now a certainty.

Never before have you had the plan, skills, ability, mindset, techniques, strategies, tactics and confidence to conquer obesity in your life so that you can create the lifestyle of your dreams.

You now have those skills, the power, and the mojo. Use them. Perfect them. Celebrate your transformation.

**Weight Loss for Wimps™
Success Step Ten**

> **<u>Attitude</u>**: I acknowledge that I have been unnecessarily fearful of experiencing real hunger.
>
> I now understand that hunger pangs are normal and that I will likely experience them on a daily basis during my weight loss phase and during my future maintenance program.
>
> **<u>Skills</u>**: I know how to distinguish between real hunger and fake (phantom) hunger.
>
> I will adopt the self-talk *Hunger Is Good™ Mindset* when dealing with real hunger.
>
> I will incorporate high fiber and high-protein foods into my diet, where appropriate, to help combat hunger. I will also use high

volume, low calorie soups and salads in my meal planning.

I will implement the *I Learn™* and *I Love Good Food™* techniques for dealing with fake hunger along with diversion, distraction, movement, activity.

<u>Action</u>: Recalibrate your body and mind to experiencing real hunger for a day. Do not eat anything after breakfast, until the evening meal. Make notes in your personal journal each hour during the day to record your hunger levels (strong, weak, none) and how long any hunger pangs lasted. Drink plenty of water or tea during this test.

Review your notes after dinner to detect any patterns. How many incidents of hunger? How long did they last? Did you survive? Big deal or not a big deal?

PART THREE

FOOD
EAT, EAT, EAT!

CHAPTER ELEVEN

THE BEST WEIGHT LOSS DIET IN THE WORLD

NOW THE FUN starts. You get to pick the eating program that will make you healthy, sexy and thin, for life! Isn't that exciting?!

Remember my pledge to you earlier - with 25,000 diet books out there, the last thing you need me to do is create another one. Choosing a plan, program or style of eating is something very personal and a decision <u>you</u> need to make.

Having said that, the easy thing for me to do would be to just tell you to go find a commercial diet program you like and implement that choice. More on this subject below.

But that's not where I'm coming from. I'm not out to just sell you a book on losing weight. I'm trying to change your thinking, change your habits and therefore change your life *permanently* so that you become healthy and thin with wholesome, real foods that you love.

My goal is to get you off the Western diet style of eating that has been so destructive to our collective health. You must do this first for yourself, and then teach your other family members, especially your children.

That's my goal, and I'm drawing a line in the sand for you, too! Learn, accomplish and then teach. Let's work together to change the world, agreed?

Commercial Diet Programs

Certainly, there are several well known programs that have been very successful (commercially, meaning many repeat customers) for many years and for some people have worked well. These would include names like Jenny Craig®, Nutrisystem®, and Medifast®.

I never recommend these programs to my clients because in general, they continue to promote the consumption of Western diet foods (although in smaller quantities), or they offer their own brand of foods from unknown sources, which are generally of low to mediocre quality. I could go on and on, but you get the picture.

Nevertheless, if one of these programs is particularly appealing to you or convenient, I say go for it. Just make the transition back to "real food" as soon as you can.

The only well known diet programs that I will recommend to people are the South Beach Diet® and Weight Watchers®. This is because these two generally promote a healthy blend of the three main macronutrient groups (proteins, carbohydrates and fats) that you cook yourself with real food. And South Beach in particular teaches you to avoid the Western diet (discussed further below), the food selections quickly stabilize and improve your blood chemistry (sugars, fats and hormones), and is very easy to follow.

The South Beach Diet® helps you make a good transition and sets you on the path towards healthy eating habits. As an additional bonus, you don't have to weigh food or count calories - yeah!!!!

The Evils of Our Western Diet
Every good book needs a villain.

Sure, I've introduced you to the all-star players who are out to stop your progress at every turn - excuses, emotional eating, stress and hunger. These guys are the enforcers, the street thugs that are out on the corner every day.

But pull back the curtain, and you have the real power behind the game – the ***Western Diet.***

Author Michael Pollan in his book, *In Defense of Food* , refers to the Western diet as the "elephant in the room" nobody wants to talk about when discussing diet and health. I also like to think of it as the "800-lb gorilla."

There are several definitions of the "Western Diet" depending on the specific context. My definition would be as follows:

The Western diet refers to foods that have been highly processed, treated or manufactured by an industrialized system (typically involving chemical additions) designed to enhance the ability to transport, store and ultimately sell the food for profit.

The end result is a wide variety of great tasting but low nutrient food types that are characterized by some combination of low to non-existent fiber content, high salt content, high sugar content (especially high fructose corn syrup - HFCS), high calorie content, high in nitrates and MSG preservatives and oftentimes, containing highly processed oils (hydrogenated, trans fat oils i.e. corn, safflower and soybean oils).

Western Diet Food Types

Deli meats*	Various crackers	Chips	Cakes
Pies	Pastries	Jellies	Fruit juices
Ketchup	Mayonnaise	Ice cream	Cheeses
Canned soups	French fries	Fried foods	White breads
White pasta	White rice	White flour	Coffee creamers
Candy	Pizzas	Breakfast cereals	Pancake mixes
Cookies	Corn tortillas	Colas & soft drink**	Latte's

*deli meats include ham, pastrami, bologna, hot dogs, sausages, bacon
**HFCS colas, soft drinks and coffees are the largest source of our calories (20%)

All of these products are cheap, have a long shelf life, are easily transportable and are readily available at fast-food restaurants worldwide. These are the *classic junk foods* that clog our grocery store shelves. But they also clog our arteries and mess up our blood sugar and hormone levels.

You need to also include in the Western diet description the industrialized beef, pork, fish, and poultry farms, feedlots and factories which force feed their animals with government subsidized (cheap) corn and soy based products and fill their veins with growth hormones, antibiotics and digestive enzymes to keep them plump and alive long enough to harvest at a profit.

What started out several centuries ago as a great idea to take food from an area of great abundance, then transport/store and deliver to people in areas of lesser abundance, has evolved into a worldwide food creation and distribution system that is literally making us fat and sick.

I am fully supportive of technology, industrialization, progress and capitalism.

But I draw the line when I discover that our food system is causing us great harm. The evidence is now well known and irrefutable. To quote Dr. Pollan:

> *"The Western diet is the story of the most radical change to the way humans eat since the discovery of agriculture.... the fact is that the chronic diseases that now kill most of us (obesity, diabetes, heart disease and cancer) can be traced directly to the industrialization of our food: The rise of highly processed foods and refined grains; the use of chemicals to raise plants and animals in huge monocultures; the superabundance of cheap calories of sugar and fat produced by modern agriculture; and the narrowing of the biological diversity of the human diet to a tiny handful of staple crops, notably wheat, corn and soy."*

The decisive evidence for me is the several studies of various native, isolated populations from around the world (China, Iceland, Greece, Australia, India, Peru) who have thrived on extremely limited diets (some high fat, others low fat, or high carb, low carb, all meat, all plants – *traditional, natural, whole food diets*) and have thrived in the total absence of our Western diseases of obesity, diabetes, heart disease and cancer.

But bring any of these people into the modern, industrialized world and they quickly begin getting the same diseases we all get now. It's not genetics; it's our Western diet and lifestyle which rewards conveniences and inactivity.

As Dr. Pollan concludes, *"...the human animal is well adapted to a great many different diets. The Western diet, however, is not one of them."*

What is it about the Western diet that is so terribly wrong?

No one knows for sure but there are several theories out there that seem to make sense. My interpretation:

The Western diet results in obesity and malnutrition (resulting in a variety of diseases) because it lacks a consistent and balanced supply of the major macronutrients (protein, fats, carbohydrates), the micronutrients (minerals, vitamins), and it is especially deficient in fiber. In addition, it contains an oversupply of certain sugars, salts and fats that cause insulin, estrogen and many other hormones to become significantly out of balance.

Remember that our modern Western diet is a new invention in terms of our hunter-gatherer ancestral history. White sugar as we know it today was only first introduced in 1812 and was not widely available until the early Twentieth Century.

 It turns out that the physiology of our body is not well adapted to these recent "improvements" in our food supplies.

So, what's the answer? Regress back to our aboriginal lifestyle?

In a sense, yes.

Cut the crap and burn the fat. Remember that?

The "crap" that you must cut is the Western diet and all the fake foods that go along with it. That's it… declare war and eliminate them immediately, if not sooner!

Go on a war path to clean out your kitchen and get rid of all the junk food, once and for all. If it's not in your cupboard, you won't be tempted to eat it.

Here's a tip… what I did was to train my brain so that when I saw junk food that I could no longer eat, I just said to myself…"*I don't eat that crap anymore!*"

I guarantee that if you did nothing else but eliminate all that junk food and liquid calories from your diet, the excess fat on your body will melt off very, very quickly, like an ice cube on a hot summer day.

"But, if I cut out all the crap, what is left for me to eat?"

In Search of the Perfect Diet
What is left is an almost endless variety of fruits, vegetables, beans, nuts, nonfat dairy, whole grains and meat/poultry/fish/seafood that can be combined into the most delicious and fulfilling meals you can imagine. Healthy, nutrition-packed real, natural, whole foods that allow your body to heal from the evils of the Western diet.

The issue at this point is to decide the style of eating that will accomplish all of your goals.

Let's come up with some general criteria for selecting an eating style or program that will accomplish our health and weight loss goals, and make us happy!

Here are the criteria I use (your choices may be slightly different):

- Great tasting food
- No deprivation; fulfilling meals; minimizes but not eliminates hunger
- Limited or no calorie counting (tracking "points" is fine)
- Limited or no weighing or measuring of food (just eyeball measurements)
- Provides for a caloric deficit
- Healthy and nutritious foods, not just calorie restrictive
- Flexibility in food choices to allow great variety
- Long-term eating plan rather than a short-term "diet"
- Easy food preparation
- Can be adapted to personal and cultural preferences

The "personal and cultural preferences" criterion is important because many people have specific personal and or cultural reasons for eating or not eating certain foods. For example, people who are vegetarian, vegan, or those who desire a kosher or gluten-free regime. Other styles could include the general categories of Mexican, Spanish, French, German, Italian, Japanese, Chinese, Asian, or Mediterranean as well as distinct regional and local food preferences.

It sounds like a difficult task to choose the perfect eating program that takes into account all of the above factors. But, it's really quite simple when you think about it.

"Everything should be made as simple as possible, but not simpler." ~ Albert Einstein

The *Perfect Diet* for you requires only three things: (1) you need to pick real, natural, whole foods that you love (or at least like); (2) prepare them with the appropriate oils, spices and seasonings to enhance their flavor; and (3) eat them according to a set of rules or guidelines that promote the desired health and weight loss goals you've established for yourself.

Again, I'm not going to spell out a diet program with recipes for you. There are plenty of resources out there if you need help with items (1) and (2).

The final leg of our Perfect Diet tripod is the eating rules or guidelines. Let's work on that next.

10 Abraham Lincoln Eating Rules™

Abraham Lincoln was the 16th President of the United States, until his untimely death at the age of 56 by assassination in 1865. I have chosen him to use as a model for eating rules for several reasons.

Lincoln was a tall, slender man and reportedly very strong (a good wrestler). He loved all types of animals and apparently did not include much meat in his diet (a good rule but not a deal-breaker).

I use him primarily to signify a time in our human history when our eating habits were simple, our daily physical activity level was much higher and most importantly, obesity, heart disease, diabetes and cancer were very rare. We should all strive to create a similar lifestyle.

Rule 1 – take Abraham Lincoln with you when you go grocery shopping. Do not buy any food items that *he* would not recognize. That means you will shop primarily along the outer aisles of

188

the store for vegetables, fruit, eggs, milk, and a variety of meat/poultry/fish/seafood items; you will generally stay out of the center aisles where all the junk food is typically located.

Rule 2 – eat wild, grass fed or pastured animal protein only; use meat/fish as a side dish, not the main course.

Rule 3 – control portions by never, never eating a second helping of any food item (except salad).

Rule 4 – include protein, carbohydrates and fats with every meal; do not follow one of the fad diets which usually eliminate carbs or fats.

Rule 5 – never skip breakfast; even if it's just a fruit smoothie or a low calorie breakfast bar. This is the only meal you need to eat even when you are not feeling real hunger - it's that important.

Rule 6 – do not eat unless you are hungry; stop eating when you are no longer hungry; plan to eat five to six small meals per day including healthy snacks

Rule 7 – eat very slowly, concentrating on the fabulous taste, smell and texture of each bite; put your eating utensils down between bites.

Rule 8 – include foods high in fiber with each meal; a food rich in fiber, such as oatmeal, fruits and vegetables have a low calorie density and significantly extend the feeling of fullness.

Rule 9 – drink clean, clear water at a rate of about half a cup per hour, every hour you are awake. Eliminate tap water if you can afford to purchase or make filtered water. Add green or white tea and coffee as desired.

Rule 10 – create a caloric deficit each and every day by managing your calorie intake and increasing your calorie consumption through increased body movement and lean muscle building exercises (Chapter 13).

This last rule, creating a calorie deficit, is the centerpiece of the *Weight Loss for Wimps™ System* – without burning more calories than you take in, you won't lose weight. Let's get clear on this issue.

How Many Calories Should I Eat?
The answer to this extremely important question can get very complicated very quickly. This is

because technically, it involves a person's sex, age, height, current weight, activity level, and baseline or resting metabolic rate. The desired rate of weight loss is also an important factor.

I like to keep things simple and straightforward, so let's skip all the technical stuff and go directly to the answer. Assuming you would like a slightly more aggressive rate of weight loss (I suggest a target of about 10-12 lbs per month; 2.5-3 lbs/week), I would recommend the following:

Women: 1100-1300 calories per day
Men: 1500-2000 calories per day

An alternative approach is based on your current weight: 8 calories per pound of bodyweight. For example, a 250 lb person would calculate at 2000 calories per day (250 x 8 = 2000).

Are these the right numbers for you?

The only way to find out for sure is to closely monitor your calorie intake for a week and then measure your results. Did you lose 2-3 lbs or not?

If you didn't, simply cut your intake back a little (look at your natural carbs like brown rice, whole wheat bread and cereals) and increase your exercise a little. With a little practice, you can quickly learn to "eyeball" your plate to calculate the approximate calories and make adjustments on the fly.

Remember, as you lose more and more weight, your body will need less and less calories to maintain its current weight. That means for example, if you were losing weight at 250 lbs and 2000 calories per day, when you reach 220 lbs, you probably won't lose weight at 2000 calories (1750 may be about right). You get the idea - monitor and adjust as needed for your situation.

A note of caution: do not get too aggressive with your calorie cutting for more than three weeks at a time. For example, if your calculated deficit is 1500 calories per day and you want to do 1200 calories per day, don't stay at this level for more than three weeks. This is because your body will go into "starvation mode" to conserve energy/fat by slowing down your metabolism, regardless of your intake and calorie usage level.

Every three weeks, bounce your calories back up to the 1700 to 2000 calorie level for a couple of days. This will stimulate your metabolism and cycle it out of going into starvation mode. You might consider taking this opportunity to use the *No Fear*™ cheating technique you learned earlier (Chapter Six) to satisfy any of your cravings.

The Best Diet in the World and the Perfect Diet are one and the same…an eating program selected and designed by *you to meet your* specific tastes, health and weight loss goals.

You are ready now. Choose the day that will be your *Transformation Day* – the first day of your new life and new lifestyle.

Implement and Celebrate!

In the next chapter, I'll show you how I put it all together into a Forrest Gump simple program that allowed me to lose 88 lbs.

Weight Loss for Wimps™
Success Step Eleven

> **Attitude**: I now understand that the Western diet is no longer acceptable in my life.

I acknowledge that eliminating junk food from my house and diet must become a top priority that I will implement immediately.

When I see my (formerly) favorite junk food, I will say to myself, *"I don't eat that crap anymore!"*

<u>**Skills**</u>: I will adopt an eating style that will incorporate clean, fresh vegetables, fruits, lean proteins and whole grains.

I will study, memorize and implement the *10 Abraham Lincoln Eating Rules™*, into my life immediately.

I will estimate my daily calorie intake needs and make necessary adjustments based on actual results. I will record my food consumption in my personal daily log. A free *Weight Loss for Wimps™ Daily Journal* (including a daily food log) is available at: http://www.wimpdailyjournal.com

<u>**Action**</u>: Choose an eating style that is compatible with your personal beliefs, philosophy and family values.

Begin researching and collecting recipes for foods that you really like. Make a shopping list for the next week and go shopping.

Decide which day (today?) will be your *Transformation Day* – the first day of your new life and new lifestyle - mark it on your calendar and record it in your personal journal.

Implement and Celebrate!

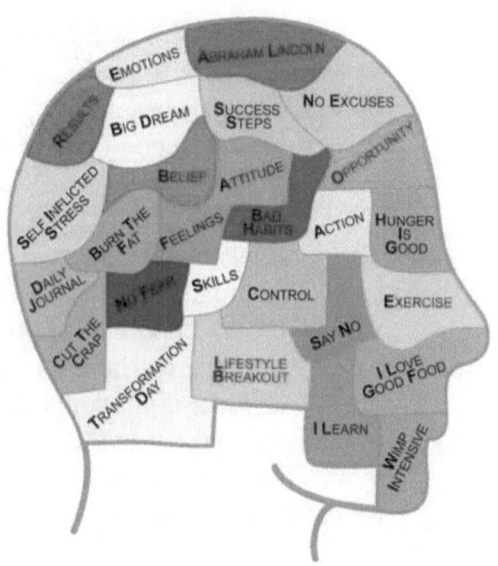

CHAPTER TWELVE

THE SIMPLE DIET
THAT SAVED MY LIFE AND
ALLOWED ME TO LOSE 88 LBS

LIFE IS NOT a Bowl of Cherries
When I returned home to Costa Rica after three long weeks at fat camp and having lost 17 lbs, I was pumped up beyond belief. I had the opportunity to focus 100% of my thoughts and energy on me, and was ready to face the day-to-day challenges in the real world. Or so I thought…

Things started off great. My wife loves to cook so I handed her a stack of recipes I had picked up at fat camp. I can barely boil water so I was thankful I was in good hands with her cooking skills.

That first week was fantastic. My wife, my dog and I were up and out the door for our power walk at 0 dark hundred every morning. We would then hike up the hill to the swimming pool (Abby, the dog, would do a couple of laps to cool off) and on up the hill to the outside gymnasium for weight lifting. Then back home for coffee and breakfast.

Exactly one week after my return home, disaster struck; my wife had an accident that changed both of our lives forever.

Long story short, she fractured the top of her lower leg bone (tibia) that required a titanium plate with six screws. It was a very, very bad break. She was in the hospital for 5 days and then in a wheelchair for the next three months. She has since recovered fully after intense physical therapy and is doing fine. She will eventually need a full knee replacement, but we'll deal with that in the future.

The whole affair was very intense for me too, both emotionally and physically. Of course, I had to immediately shift the focus of my energy to taking care of my wife. This entailed doing many things I had never done before in our 30+ years of marriage... bedpans, administering shots into her stomach for 28 days (anti-coagulant), taking her up and down fairly steep ramps, doing the laundry, grocery shopping and cooking (sort of).

The good part of all of this was that I was able to keep eating reasonably healthy meals and, because of all the additional body movement expended attending to her, I significantly increased my daily exercise and calorie expenditures. I also learned some new housekeeping skills (laundry, how to operate the dishwasher, shopping and a little cooking) and now have no excuses for not helping out!

Within another couple of months, another tragedy hit us - my wife's mother suddenly passed away back in California. With all this trauma in our lives, we made the decision to return to the U.S. permanently. Our four year adventure in Costa Rica had been fun and exciting, but it was time to go back home.

In spite of these setbacks, I continued dropping weight rather quickly. Sure, it would have been easy to just say the heck with it, and revert back to my old eating habits and couch potato lifestyle. But I was feeling better than I had in years, so I was not giving up.

I learned a long time ago that bad stuff happens to good people. I'm pretty sure that bad things have happened to you and probably much worse than what I just described. The trick of course, is to not let these events destroy you.

The mindset is simple enough…

> *"These things happened to me (recently or back when) and they were horrible. I would not wish them to happen to my worst enemy. But I have to accept that it*

*happened (life can be a
bitch) and move on. I must
focus on enjoying the
present and looking forward
to the future."*

I stuck with it and made the transition to a permanent lifestyle change that has been with me now for going on four years. You can do the same thing!

Simple Healthy Meals - For Dummies Like Me!

I don't cook (except on the grill) but I take responsibility for what goes in my mouth. Well, I now cook a little and I'm learning more as I watch the Food Channel. But I insist on only two things; simple to prepare and healthy.

I promised you I wasn't going to get into recipes. But I would like to at least describe some of the meals I ate while losing weight and the overall approach I take to eating. In addition to the *10 Abraham Lincoln Eating Rules*™ discussed in the last chapter, here are some of my personal rules:

- As I mentioned previously, I really don't like to count calories. That is, I don't keep detailed records. However, I do

199

keep an approximate running total in my head so as to not totally blow it. That requires me to read labels, know serving sizes and to look up the calorie count of my most common foods. I try to keep my daily calorie count to 1200 or below when I'm in the weight loss mode, but not lower than 800 calories (these numbers are not necessarily good for you).

- I avoid "white" - white rice, white bread, white flour products; I substitute brown i.e. whole wheat in limited quantities

- I limit my meal choices to just a few that I enjoy and stick with those. I found this approach to be very successful, although it can be a little boring at times. The advantage is you know it is working; it simplifies shopping and meal preparation and removes the mystery of researching new recipes.

For example, for breakfast I eat either a bowl of steel cut oat meal with a splash of skim milk, a half a cup of blueberries and Splenda® brown sugar; or I substitute Shredded Wheat or Kashi® Crunch. Total calories about 270 on the high end (I round it to 300 for ease of addition). This meal is also high in soluble fiber and antioxidants, but also contains protein, carbohydrates and a variety of other essential vitamins. And, it is filling!

For morning and afternoon snacks, I will have a handful of raw walnuts, raisins or a cup fresh fruit like cantaloupe or an apple. I try to keep the snacks to about 100 to 150 calories.

Lunch is typically a quick sandwich and some fruit; I like the Oroweat Sandwich Thins™ (100 calories and 5 grams of fiber), shaved turkey breast (or chicken), a slice of low fat cheese with a bit of mustard. Add in a handful of grapes and I have a filling lunch that contains about 350 calories.

Dinner is much more varied and a bit more challenging from a calorie counting standpoint. This is because my wife typically prepares the dinner meal and I have to pay attention to her recipes and particularly the portion sizes. Generally, this is the only meal we share because we each do our own thing for breakfast and lunch.

Here's the basic approach I take for dinner:
- 1/3 of the plate for vegetables

- 1/3 of the plate for whole grains (brown rice) **_or_** legumes (beans)
- 1/3 of the plate for protein i.e. beef, pork, chicken, turkey, eggs or fish

Notice a few important points about this "eyeball" approach…

1) Two thirds of the meal plate is plant based; vegetables, whole grains and or legumes

2) Only one third is available for protein

3) Whole grains and legumes are limited to reduce the overall caloric load of the meal; generally it's either whole grain or beans although a mixture of the two is fine as long as you restrict the portion size to third of your plate.

With portion control, this approach to the dinner will produce a meal of about 375 to 450 calories.

Shhhhhh! Still want recipes? Go to the home page at www.weightloss4wimps.com and on the right margin, you will find a box where you can download some great, low calorie single-pot and comfort food recipes - awesome!

Portion Control Made Easy
Controlling the serving size or portions is really all about the *volume* of food you put into your

body. And it is critical to the "eyeball approach" to calorie counting. Don't think that just because you are limiting your protein for example, you can load up on everything else. Think about how many overweight "vegetarians" that you know. Anyway, here's my basic technique:

- I never go for seconds, except for vegetables

- I limit whole grains and beans to an ice cream scoop or half a baseball sized portion

- I limit my protein to a deck of cards portion (about 4 ounces)

Exercise - Completing the Trifecta
I ultimately figured out the mental aspects of weight control i.e. the process of dealing with excuses, dealing with hunger, dealing with stress and with emotions...

I developed a sound approach to eating such that I was consuming healthy and nutritious foods but in portions that gave me a chance to create a caloric deficit...

I needed to stick with an exercise program that "guaranteed" that I created a caloric deficit each and every day.

The approach that worked for me was (and continues today) as follows:

- I walk six days a week for about 45 minutes to 1 hour each day (about 2.5 to 3 miles)

- Three days a week, in addition to the walking, I lift weights to increase (and maintain) my lean muscle mass

- In addition to these more programmed events, I look for opportunities to move my body more frequently throughout the day…anything to keep moving and avoid sitting around and doing nothing. This could be playing a round of golf, walking around the mall, working in the yard; even taking my Harley for a ride is better than nothing!

These are the attitudes and methods that have worked well for me. You are different and therefore will need to adopt these elements into your life in perhaps, a different way. That is to be expected and encouraged.

The main idea is to break out of your current "unhealthy lifestyle" and develop a new and improved version of <u>you</u>.

The next section of this book, I call "Rocket Fuel" because these are the things that will take you to the next level and ensure your weight loss success. These include more information on exercise, the importance of monitoring your progress and finally, the concept of public accountability.

Buckle up… here we go!

Weight Loss for Wimps™
Success Step Twelve

<u>Attitude</u>: Evaluate the attitudes that I have adopted to supplement my eating style and see if any are appropriate for you.

<u>Skills</u>: I will develop a set of portion control rules to insure that I will never over eat and will strive to always create a caloric deficit

Action: Record in your journal any supplemental attitudes that you will incorporate in your eating rules. I will document my portion control rules and will diligently follow them at every meal

PART FOUR

ROCKET FUEL
FOR
LIFESTYLE BREAKOUT
SUCCESS

CHAPTER THIRTEEN

EXERCISE:
GET THAT BUTT MOVING!

MY GOAL IN THIS chapter is to convince you to forever overcome your basic desire to continue your couch potato lifestyle. I know, it's a most difficult task but I <u>will</u> succeed!

What do you need to get started?

You need a swift kick in the butt, that's what you need! And you may need a personal trainer and/or a coach which will be discussed in the next chapter.

But most of all, you need to be convinced that getting your butt out the door (or to the gym) <u>*and loving it*</u> is your new lifestyle.

It takes a little practice to permanently adopt an exercise routine into your life. But trust me, you <u>will</u> get to the point where you actually look forward to your workouts. Sounds weird right now, but that's only because it hasn't been a part of your life for a long while, if ever.

The benefits will blow your mind:
- You will feel better
- You will look better
- Your health will improve dramatically
- You will lose weight much, much quicker
- Bonus – your sex life will improve!

The approach I am going to take is to (a) remove any and all excuses; (b) shame you; (c) piss you off; (d) motivate you; (e) show you the simple/minimalist path; (f) show you a slightly more comprehensive path; (g) encourage you!

Let's get started with excuses.

I Hate To Exercise!
Really... you *hate* to exercise?

What happened?

You loved to "exercise" when you were a kid and played in the street until the streetlights went on.

You loved to "exercise" when you were a teenager and couldn't wait to play baseball, basketball, football, tennis or soccer at school.

You loved to "exercise" when you were a young adult of college age and played on the school team, intramurals, and fraternity or on a local city league team; or when you served your country in the military.

You loved to "work out" when you played professionally in the MLB, NFL, NHL or NBA.

What happened is; you got a job, started a career, started a family, lost a job, got injured, retired and/or otherwise let life get in the way of an active, healthy lifestyle. That's the sanitized version.

What really happened is you ***got lazy*** and have created a series of *good sounding excuses* to justify your laziness to yourself:

- "I'm so frickin' busy at work just trying to survive my dipstick boss…"
- "I've got such a long commute, I just can't find the time…"
- "I've got to spend my free time with the wife and kids…"
- "I can't afford to buy barbells/weights or join a gym…"
- "I blew out my knee and can't jog…"

Whatever, whatever, blah, blah, blah… (see Chapter Seven on *Dealing With Excuses*)

In the meantime, you've gotten fat (maybe even obese), your sex life is in radio silence mode, you're too embarrassed to go to your class reunion, if you're single you can't get a date off a calendar, etc. And that's the good news!

Hopefully, this doesn't apply to you but the bad news is that you may have developed a variety of health issues directly tied to your obesity and lifestyle (i.e. Type 2 diabetes, heart disease).

You *can* lose weight without exercise. But here's the deal; your weight loss will be very, very slow and you will have little room for error with your daily caloric intake. Overshoot your burn rate and you will not lose any weight, or worse still you will gain weight.

What we want to do here is add **Rocket Fuel** to your fat loss effort so it's done quickly and with gusto and that is accomplished with exercise.

But wait - maybe you need a little more motivation. Let's see.

Oh No… You've Got "Man-Boobs?!"
If you've got man-boobs, you're in famous
company with the likes of actors Jack
Nicholson, Jack Black, John Travolta and ex-
athletes George Foreman, Charles Barkley,
David Wells, Billy Joe Tolliver, Bill Parcells,
Rex Ryan, for example.

Do you think Jack Nicholson, with his now
famous "man-boobs" *can handle the <u>truth</u>?*
Check him out here: <u>http://bit.ly/obv938</u>

Yes, these famous celebrities can still attract a
crowd of fawning fans because of their fame
and money. But I can guarantee you that these
folks would love to have their sleek, fit bodies
back so they could strut their stuff with
confidence in public. The exception is the
actor/comedian Jack Black, who claims *"…I am
proud of my man-boobs."* Yeah, right.

For most men, this is your worst nightmare!

Although there is a medical condition called
gynecomastia (cause uncertain), in most cases
the condition is due to hormone imbalance
(estrogen/testosterone) caused by poor diet, lack
of exercise and the resulting obesity.

If man-boobs are an issue with you, don't worry; the solution is easy:

Cut the crap and burn the fat with <u>exercise</u>!

Poof… the man-boobs will disappear almost instantly.

Why do I bring this up? So you will stop kidding yourself. If this is a problem in your life, it requires your immediate attention.

Oh… one more thing…

I have done extensive, detailed research/interviews with women at the most popular nightclubs all across the country and around the world (don't I wish!)…hold the press… the results are in…

Women find beer bellies, fat butts and man-boobs to be among the most unattractive features on men

Ok, that's enough - I've got you pissed off, upset, self-conscious but hopefully **motivated**! Maybe, just maybe, this is the ***Tipping Point*** you've been missing but desperately need in order to make that lifestyle change and lose weight successfully!

213

It's time to man up and get your butt moving.
Or if you're among the vast and expanding
group of smart women reading this book, it's
time to *cowgirl up* as we say in Texas and talk
to your man about his man-boobs; and get *your*
butt moving too!

Yeah - that's what I'm talking about!

Can You Spare Fifteen Minutes for a Workout?

I'm going to totally eliminate the most popular
excuse for not exercising…

"I'm too busy; I just don't have the time…"

My thought: Boo-Frickin'-Hoo!

If you can't find 15 minutes then you need to do
some serious priority adjustments in your life.
You need to *simplify your life*; this is a self-
inflicted wound you have created.

News flash: just got a hot tip from one of my
personal trainer buds on Twitter: How to fit
workouts into a busy schedule – (a) get up early
and (b) go to bed earlier!

I'm going to show you an exercise routine that meets your every need and otherwise meets the following criteria:

- It only takes *15 minutes* out of your day, three times a week (45 minutes a week)

- Does not require you to purchase any equipment, weights, etc.

- Does not require you to join a local gymnasium (but you may want to)

- A variation can be done at home, at work, indoors, outdoors or at a gym

- Will help you burn fat like a blow torch and maximize your caloric deficit!

- Is touted as the "world's more effective exercise for long-term weight loss and health"

Really... a 15 minute workout is going to do it for me? Yep, and I didn't just make this up! It's a protocol that is similar to that of several well-known exercise guru's - names like Tim Ferris, Matt Furey, Craig Ballantyne, and Dr. Al Sears MD, to name a few.

The basic protocol is this:

Move your body *very intensively* for short bursts of time (10-30 seconds),
Slow down and catch your breath for two minutes,
Repeat.

That's it - it doesn't get any simpler than that!

I call this basic technique the *Wimp Intensive*™

Wimp Intensive™ *Workout Protocol*
Before we get into the specifics of the workout, a very, very important word of caution is in order. This style of exercise is very hard on your body, particularly at the beginning. (Again, check with your physician before starting this or any other exercise program). This means you can be in great danger of **injury** i.e. muscle tear, ligament/tendon injury, hamstring, or Achilles tear. Remember, your body probably hasn't seen this level of exertion in many moons!

Proceed with great caution:

Start Very Slow and Gradually Build Up Your Speed and Repetitions

I will be introducing you to a total of six (6) types of intensive exercise. If you are in generally poor to fair physical condition at the moment, you will need to start with either the walk or pool protocol with only four (4) repetitions.

A word about repetitions – starting out you will only do four (4) repetitions i.e. four (4) spurts of 15-30 seconds each, followed by a rest/slow walk of two (2) minutes. Over a few weeks or months (depending on how you feel) gradually add more repetitions up to a maximum of eight (8).

Again, you are only doing this workout 2-3 times per week to give your body periods of regeneration between intense exertions.

Now, a word about speed or intensity – firstly, you will need to start each workout with a warm up period of about two to five minutes. This can consist of a brisk walk and some stretching; this is very important to prevent injury!

Second, as you begin the first rep, you will only need to go at about 25% of full speed; the remaining reps should be at about 50% of your max speed.

You want to be "huffing and puffing" at the end of each repetition but don't want to burn out after the first two or three bursts!

Let's go through the various options that you may choose:

1. *The Wimp Walk*

This assumes you are outside (sidewalks are free!) but actually could be done anywhere (i.e. at an indoor shopping mall). With this protocol, you simply do your 15-30 second high intensity bursts at a *fast walk*. Walk as fast as you comfortably can, typically at about a 4.5 miles per hour pace. After you finish the burst, slow to crawl or about 1.5 miles per hour while you catch your breath for two (2) minutes - but do not stop walking. Rinse and repeat three (3) more times and you're done! In less than 15 minutes!

To make this work out even better, do this on a hill that you can walk up. This will increase the intensity and help build up your all important quad muscles.

2. *The Wimp Sprint*

With this protocol, you simply do your 15-30 second bursts at a sprint; do this as a 55 yard (50 meter) or 110 yard (100 meter) dash depending

on your strength/endurance level. You can start
out at a slow run of five (5) mph and ramp up to
about eight (8) mph (and higher as you improve
your fitness level).

Again, you want to be out of breath and huffing
and puffing but then be able to recover within
the 2 minute slow walk period.

Similar to the walk protocol, your workout will
be improved if you can find an outside area with
a gentle slope (5-7%).

3. *The Wimp Treadmill*
This option is one of my favorites but does
require that you either own a home treadmill or
join a local gym/fitness center. The reason I like
the treadmill is that you can quickly adjust your
speed and the elevation within seconds. Plus,
most of the professional models have a built in
timer display to easily track your duration.

And doing the workout indoors is a great option
when the weather is either "too damn hot" or
"too damn cold" outside which, in north Texas,
is half of the year!

After a 2-5 minute warm up walk, just crank up
the elevation to about 5-7 degrees (eventually
up to 15 degrees) and the speed up to about 4.5

mph for a fast walk or 5-8 mph for a jog/run. As you approach the end of your burst, simply lower the speed down to one and a half (1.5) mph and then lower the elevation back down to zero; catch your breath for two (2) minutes, then repeat.

4. *The Wimp Stairs*
This protocol is designed primarily for those poor souls who are (a) stuck working in an office building and (b) have access to at least two (2) flights of stairs (one floor level). This is also designed for those who claim they don't have time to work out cuz they work too much - gotcha again!

Get your 15-30 second burst by walking or jogging up at least one floor level; catch your breath for 2 minutes (go down stairs or keep moving) and repeat. Out of breath yet?!

The gym I go to has a second floor so I am able to do this there for a great add-on workout. Of course, you can also use a *Stairmaster*™ or similar in the gym.

5. *The Wimp Pool*
I do this workout with my wife because she has knee issues and we both enjoy swimming at the pool.

A 30 second burst, any stroke you chose, is typically one length of a standard Olympic sized pool. After the first burst, take a two (2) minute rest (keep moving while you rest), swim hard and fast then repeat for the remaining repetitions. You will be "huffing and puffing" which is the idea! Excellent workout alternative for those with joint problems or other limitations.

See how simple a great workout can be?

The best advice I can give you on the workout is to keep it *intense* and try to change your routine frequently so that you use all five (5) protocols in order to use different muscles and also to prevent boredom!

But let me add a little commentary to the benefits discussed above. This simple, intensive workout can be deceiving because it is over so quickly. Let me assure you this - give it two weeks minimum and you will be amazed with the results!

The added benefits that this style of workout brings to the table include (a) expanding your lungs capacity; (b) blows out the poisons hiding deep in your lungs; (c) dramatically improves your heart muscle and its circulation; (d) builds lean muscle tissue in your legs; (e) speeds up your baseline resting metabolism for up to 48 hours thus increasing your overall daily caloric burn rate.

In short, it is ideal for a weight loss program and a significant plus to a healthy lifestyle.

Now, if you are so inclined and can "squeeze in a little more time in your busy schedule," let's add another 30 minutes of weight training to _really_ add rocket fuel to your weight loss program.

Wimp Weight Lifting
The intellectual concept about why weight lifting a.k.a. resistance training is necessary for increasing the speed of weight loss is simple: as you add lean muscle cells/tissue to your body, you (a) increase the overall resting metabolism rate and (b) you have more cells in your body competing for a fixed or limited supply of energy. Translation: you burn stored fat!

Imagine your body right now, as you are reading this. Let's say for discussion purposes that your body is composed of 100,000 cells. Each cell requires certain nutrients to maintain

222

itself and consumes a certain amount of energy (glucose) as it goes about its daily business.

As you go about lifting weights, in a certain way as discussed below, your body takes raw nutrients from your digestive/circulatory system and manufactures new lean muscle tissue. Let's say that over time, your body adds 10,000 new lean muscle tissue cells. You now have 10% more cells in your body (110,000) that are working for you and screaming at you 24/7 – _feed me I'm hungry!_ Your basal or resting metabolic rate has just gone up!

A variety of studies estimate that for each pound of muscle added to your body, you will burn about 50 calories more per day. Compare that with a pound of flabby fat that burns less than two (2) calories per day. Muscle is an energy hog, **_demanding 25 times more energy than fat_**. Which would you rather have?

- 10 lbs of fat will burn less that 20 calories per day
- 10 lbs of added muscle will burn 500 calories per day
- 10 lbs of added muscle will burn about 183,000 calories/year

- 183,000 calories is the amount of energy in about 53 lbs of fat

Gain 10 lbs of muscle, lose 50 lbs of fat!

Of course, I'm oversimplifying but I think you get the picture. Now, how do you go about adding lean muscle tissue to your body?

By applying the *Wimp Intensive™* philosophy to a weight training protocol.

This means you lift hard, heavy and fast; rest for one to two minutes, rinse and repeat! You work with the weight amount that allows you to complete only eight (8) reps i.e. to muscle fatigue. Do two sets of eight (8) reps at each weight station.

Note: studies have shown that eight (8) reps with heavier weight is much better at adding lean muscle tissue compared with lighter weights at 12 reps.

Work on all three sections of your body i.e. lower body, mid section and upper body. You can hit all three sections in one workout or alternate days during the week. For example, on Monday you work on the upper body, Wednesday the mid- section and Friday the lower body. Generally, try to do three to four machines/exercises for each of the three body sections.

I like to work all three body sections on each of the three days I'm in the gym during the week. I just like the variety and flexibility that this scheme allows; but chose what works best for you.

Is it necessary that I explain bench press, squats, lunges, barbell curls, lat pull down, etc.? No, I didn't think so either! If you need help in this area, talk to a trainer at the gym… they will be happy to help you.

Finally, note that studies consistently show that an intense weight lifting session of 30 minutes for example, will increase your resting metabolic rate for up to 48 hours after you complete the workout. As discussed above, this is an incredible benefit of intensive workouts making this style far superior to long and boring cardiovascular training.

Adding lean muscle tissue to your body coupled with creating a daily caloric deficit through diet and exercise is the key to rapid and healthy weight loss.

Combining the *Wimp Treadmill* for example, with the *Wimp Weight Lifting* into one 45-60 minute session will give you the fat burning blow torch that you need to drop your excess weight very quickly.

Working Out at Home
Are you one of the millions out there who don't like to get partially naked or hot and sweaty in front of strangers at a public gym? Or you just don't want to take the time to pack up and go to the nearest gym? Or you don't like the expense of joining a fitness facility?

Working out at home is the perfect solution – and it eliminates several of the well-worn, wimpy excuses at the same time!

And you really don't need to purchase any expensive exercise equipment because you can build lean muscle and get great cardio by simply using your own body weight. Of course, if you have a home gym or treadmill, clear off the clothes hanging on it and get to work!

A big help for many people is to listen to music or watch an exercise DVD while working out. If you are in that category, there are some excellent choices. I like the variety of choices available at www.beachbody.com including the

226

10-Minute Trainer, Turbo Fire and the newly released *P90X2*. Plus, you can find yourself a weight loss coach at a very modest price. Check them out!

**Weight Loss for Wimps™
Success Step Thirteen**

> **Attitude**: I acknowledge that I have not made physical activity a priority in my daily life; this behavior is no longer acceptable.
>
> My goal is to permanently leave the couch potato lifestyle behind. I have no legitimate excuse for not exercising my body on a daily basis.
>
> **Skills**: I will adjust my priorities and schedule to incorporate at least 15 minutes of intensive exercise. At a minimum, I will begin walking or swimming.
>
> I will also consider a weight lifting program because I know that it will accelerate my weight loss program and improve my fitness
>
> **Action**: Decide whether or not you are going to join a local fitness club or are going to work out at home.

Record in your daily journal the type of intensive exercise you did and how you felt afterwards. Do this every day.

CHAPTER FOURTEEN

FOR THOSE WHO WILL SETTLE FOR NOTHING LESS THAN OUTRAGEOUS SUCCESS

THIS IS THE FINAL chapter and I want to finish with a flourish! This last bit of advice will provide that little bit of extra secret sauce to produce outrageous success and will truly add *Rocket Fuel* to your weight loss journey. Strap yourself in, pay attention and prepare for blast off!

Public Accountability
Holding yourself accountable *in public* is perhaps the most powerful form of motivation of all to keep you on track with your permanent lifestyle change.

The logic in this is straightforward – you commit to change and tell your loved ones, your coach or personal trainer (or a Weight Watchers® meeting Leader) and perhaps a select few people very close to you about your plans; then you fully dedicate yourself to the new course of action and stick with it because above all else, you don't want to embarrass yourself or otherwise fail in the eyes of these people.

Just imagine in your mind's eye, the anguish of having to face these people and try to explain once again, your failure to keep your commitment to permanent change. Of course your loved ones will still love you and forgive you if you do fail, but you know the disappointment they will have.

Tell yourself, over and over, that *failure is no longer an option.* You've been down that road before and you're not going back, period.

I want you to be very selective regarding who you speak to about your lifestyle changes. Whatever you do, don't make the mistake I've seen so many people make and that is **announce your plans on Facebook** - don't do it! The truth is, many of your so-called friends, particularly on Facebook, will not be supportive and may even root for your failure. I don't know why because I'm not a psychologist! But trust me; even some of your friends in real life will try to sabotage your efforts by constantly doing little things like inviting you out for late night pizza and beer. And they will try to convince you that cheating a "little bit" won't hurt you. Of course, you have to develop the internal strength to handle social outings without cheating, but be on the lookout for saboteurs!

Take a positive leadership role and invite your friends to go with you to the gym (or a Weight Watchers® meeting, go for a walk, whatever). Don't get down in the dumps about it. Are your friends overweight? Realize that you are 57% more likely to also be overweight if you hang out with overweight friends. Obviously, that means that some of your friends likewise have poor lifestyle habits and together, you make poor choices.

In some cases you will eventually need to phase out a friend who is constantly trying to bring you back to your old habits; particularly when you start showing progress in your appearance. It's painful but sometimes necessary. If you've ever dealt with alcoholism, you know what I mean.

You are on your way to outrageous success and exceptionalism. Surround yourself with people who admire your efforts and who will help you along the way. Be social and make new friends!

The Hot, Sexy Personal Trainer
If you're going to get a personal trainer, why not get a hot, sexy one (tongue in cheek)? I like

headlines that grab your attention… have you noticed?!

I can guarantee you this - working with a good personal trainer will boost your fitness, health and weight loss results at least two-fold compared to working out by yourself. Why? Two primary reasons: (1) the "public accountability" factor discussed above; and (2) you will have a more intense and well rounded workout, specifically designed to meet your individual needs.

Once you commit to a personal trainer, you will not want to disappoint him or her by not showing up, by cancelling or by slacking off on your workout routine. It's just human nature that you will want to demonstrate to your trainer that you are committed and are making good progress.

Your fitness trainer will have had extensive training in exercise physiology and nutrition, depending on which certifications they have acquired. And they will have had experience working with clients just like you i.e. someone with a tender lower back, or knees that are painful or a shoulder that is stiff. They will be able to work with you to accommodate your specific limitations and design a program to

232

build your strength, flexibility and cardiovascular health. Plus, a trainer will generally work you much more intensely than you would on your own. Again, human nature!

A half hour session with a fitness trainer a couple of times a week would be perfect. Consider either private sessions or a group class. Also, in many communities there are fitness professionals who specialize in working with you at your home, using your equipment. There are lots of options and flexibility in finding the right person who will fit into your schedule.

Weight Loss Coaching
What about coaching? How is coaching different from a fitness trainer?

Generally speaking, a weight loss coach is someone with whom you work with over the phone discussing topics similar to those covered in this book i.e. leveraging your tipping point, dealing with excuses, hunger, emotional eating issues, etc. In other words, emphasis is placed more heavily on the mental aspects of the weight loss process rather than the physical conditioning components.

Coaching can be tailored to your specific needs, particularly if you sign up for one-on-one coaching sessions. The alternatives include weekly group sessions wherein the topics are discussed in presentation format typically followed by a question and answer session; also e-classes whereby the coaching is done entirely through email.

Here is a quote from a lady in Tennessee who posted a comment about her weight loss coaching experience:

> *"I was going to quit all together but didn't for a couple of reasons. I didn't want to let myself down and I did not want to let my coach down. I figured I'd just give up like I always do until he offered the introductory coaching session. That's when he talked to me about his program; I figured if I had someone watching over me so to speak, then I'd succeed. I usually keep my desire to lose weight to myself in case I fail; then no one can say anything to me. Now I'm telling a few close friends so I have to look them in the eye if I give up.*

Next summer I will wear a two-piece if I want; yes, even at 54!"

Public accountability, expert advice, encouragement, words of wisdom and a to-do list; that is what weight loss coaching is all about. And for many people, it is a life-changing experience that will give you that extra special edge to ensure the outrageous success that you deserve.

Interested or curious about my *Weight Loss for Wimps Coaching?*

Cool! Just send me an email and I'll let you know about the various coaching options that I have available for you; send your email to:

Coaching@weightloss4wimps.com

What's the Score – Monitoring Your Progress

One of the most important things you need to do while you're in the weight loss mode is to <u>frequently</u> weigh yourself. Remember, you can't improve what you don't measure.

There is all kinds of advice out there regarding how often you should weigh yourself.

235

Everything from never to twice daily; no kidding! There are plenty of arguments pro and con and they all have some level of validity. So it boils down to what you are comfortable with in monitoring your own progress.

My recommendation is that you weight yourself daily; first thing in the morning right after you "tinkle" (or if you're a man, "drain your radiator"!) and before you drink your first cup of coffee. Why so frequently? It's because you will start each day with your weight loss/lifestyle change front and center on your mind. A paper in the International Journal of Behavioral Nutrition and Physical Activity 2008, reported on several independent studies which show that people who weigh themselves frequently tend to lose more weight. And you want to stack the deck in your favor.

You will know instantly how you are doing, compared to yesterday. Did you lose weight or stay the same? Great, because that means you did not overeat yesterday and that you have been achieving your goal of a caloric deficit.

Did you gain weight? That may be a normal or natural variation due to water retention or other factors...or it may mean you have been overeating. Only you know how you have been doing on your compliance with your eating and exercising program. This gives you the opportunity to make immediate corrections starting <u>today</u>. Cut back a little or increase your activity a bit today (or both), and see how you do tomorrow morning.

Over a period of weeks, you will observe and learn your patterns and see how your body tends to react to your new lifestyle. And don't forget to record your daily measurements in your Journal - very important! If you haven't already done so, go to http://www.wimpdailyjournal.com and download the free *Weight Loss for Wimps™ Daily Journal.*

For those of you who are into text messaging on your mobile phone, I have the perfect solution. Just go to http://www.textweight.com

This is a very simple and efficient way to track and monitor your weight loss progress, receive reminders and tips/motivational messages daily (or on a frequency you set) and all from your mobile phone. You don't need to login to a website unless you want to see a personalized and confidential graph of your progress.

The company offers a free three month trial so how can you go wrong! Go sign yourself up today! (Note: may not be available outside the USA but they do plan to expand internationally so visit the site and let them know of your interest).

Another great option for your cell phone is to get the app from www.loseit.com where you can track your weight and also record your daily food intake/calories. Good stuff!

So here we are folks, at the end of our journey together. But your journey to outrageous weight loss success, health, fitness and happiness is just beginning. You have made the mindset adjustments, and now have all the necessary tools to work yourself through all anticipated roadblocks. And rest assured, you will encounter those nasty roadblocks each and every day. But you are ready, well prepared and you've just topped off with the *Rocket Fuel* you need to carry you all the way.

Go ahead…. Push The Button… ***BLAST OFF!***

Weight Loss for Wimps™
Success Step Fourteen

Attitude: I now understand the importance of holding myself accountable in public. It is extremely powerful, if done correctly.

I also acknowledge that I need to monitor my weight loss progress on a frequent schedule. This will allow me to make instant adjustment to my eating and physical activity levels, as necessary.

Skills: I will carefully consider with whom to share my weight loss program goals and will surround myself with very supportive people.

Action: Decide how often you will weigh yourself (at least weekly) and record your progress in your daily journal.

Decide whether or not you want to bring a fitness trainer and/or a weight loss coach into your life. At least talk to a couple of each before making a final decision.

P.S. It is now official…You are no longer a WIMP!

Be sure to let me know how you're doing - I'd love to hear from you! Send me an email to: *Kevin@weightloss4wimps.com*

Include any before and after photos too!
Visit Kevin's blog and join the conversation - your opinion is needed:

http://www.weightloss4wimps.com

APPENDIX

Master Plan

Weight Loss for Wimps™ Tools:
- *Lifestyle Breakout™ Strategy*
- *No Fear™ Cheating Technique*
- *I Learn™ To End Emotional Eating Technique*
- *I Love™ Good Food Philosophy*
- *Hunger Is Good™ Mindset*
- *10 Abraham Lincoln Eating Rules™*
- *Wimp Intensive™ Workout Protocol*

Weight Loss for Wimps™
Success Step One

<u>Attitude</u>: I know there is a price to pay to break my bad habits and I am willing to pay that price to reach my healthy weight loss goal

I am going to permanently change my eating habits and lifestyle because I want to, not because I should

<u>Skills</u>: I will get the Daily Journal at http://www.wimpdailyjournal.com and use this for my weight loss adventure

I will make a comprehensive list of all my bad habits – I know what they are!

Action: Pick two bad habits that you will focus on and eliminate *immediately*. Eliminate more as you learn the techniques to deal with negative emotions and learn to substitute healthy habits. Record these in your daily journal

Weight Loss for Wimps™
Success Step Two

Attitude: I have experienced an unpleasant tipping point in my life. I have decided that I want to resolve my weight issue now.

The glass is half full, not half empty.

Skills: I will allow myself to feel these negative emotions, recognizing that they are important and a necessary part of the process.

I will see my tipping point situation as a unique *opportunity* and a "gift" for achieving health, happiness and incredible weight loss success.

Action: Spend at least 30 minutes in quiet reflection, writing down a brief description of your tipping point(s) and noting the key negative emotions that you are feeling about it.

Think about <u>you</u>, not about others. Start thinking more about the present and your future, and less about your past. The eyes are on the **FRONT** of your head!

**Weight Loss for Wimps™
Success Step Three**

Attitude: I realize that the status quo – my habits, behaviors, the way I view myself, the way I view my future – is wimpy and unacceptable

I take full responsibility for creating my own future

Skills: I will be brutally honest with myself to discover the real reason I want to be thin – the single most important benefit to me

I will use my imagination to create an exciting, vivid vision of myself at my perfect weight. This will be my **Big Dream**.

Action: Take notes in your daily journal as you work through the <u>why</u> questions to select your biggest benefit of getting thin

Use your journal to write down the specific details of your **Big Dream**. Include feelings of empowerment, self confidence, energy and happiness. This will solidify your belief and help to make it become a reality.

**Weight Loss for Wimps™
Success Step Four**

Attitude: I give myself permission to make my health and weight loss goal <u>priority number one</u> in my life.

I am developing a healthy obsession about creating a mindset and lifestyle that will allow me to achieve my **Big Dream**

Skills: All day, every day I will reflect on the vision of my **Big Dream**

As I make my daily decisions on food choices and exercise, I will always ask myself, *"Does this move me closer to my goal or not?"*

Action: In your personal journal, write down specific changes you will commit to making in your daily routine to accommodate your new lifestyle.

Include a list of activities that you will eliminate, suspend or delegate to others to give you more time to focus on tasks related to your health and wellness.

Create a list of *new* activities that you want to do such as learning healthy meal preparation, going to the gym, riding your bicycle, taking a brisk walk, or shopping at the farmer's market.

**Weight Loss for Wimps™
Success Step Five**

Attitude: I am going to solve my weight issue once and for all

I am going "all in" to improve my health, achieve my **Big Dream** and create an extraordinary life

Skills: I will use the CDC (or similar) website to calculate my current BMI

I will use the Weight Watchers® or similar calculator to determine my long-term perfect weight goal

My short-term weight loss goal will be approximately 10 lbs per month

Action: Take a couple of photos of yourself now. Later on, you'll look at them and feel proud and amazed at your transformation.

Record your current height and weight, your starting BMI and your perfect weight goal in your daily journal.

Make a chart to record your weekly/monthly progress. Include other key measurement such as waist, thighs, and arms. You may also want to record your % weight lost on a monthly basis. This is calculated as follows: lbs lost over the month divided by starting weight at beginning of the month, times 100.

Example of Percentage Weight Loss Calculation:

Starting weight at beginning of month: 184 lbs
Weight at end of month: 174 lbs
Lbs lost: 10 lbs

10 lbs divided by 184 lbs = 0.05 X 100 = 5% weight loss

Weight Loss for Wimps™
Success Step Six

Attitude: I know the odds are against me and I've failed before. But this time is different because I'm thinking about my enemies and making plans to defeat them, *in advance*.

I am going to Anticipate, Plan and Execute

Skills: I have learned how to cheat successfully. As needed, I will implement the *No Fear™* cheating technique and use this skill with joy and without guilt. I understand this is part of the process of becoming healthy and thin.

When a cheating event occurs, I will *immediately* get back on my healthy eating program…with a smile on my face!

Action: Record in your daily journal the *No Fear™* cheating technique. Memorize the sequence so it will always be with you when needed.

Think about your current eating habits and patterns. Make notes in your journal about particular events, locations, situations or people that in retrospect, seem to trigger an overeating reaction in you. These are areas you need to work on.

Weight Loss for Wimps™
Success Step Seven

Attitude: I refuse to give up on my **Big Dream**.

I will do whatever it takes to change my lifestyle habits to get healthy and reach my perfect weight.

Skills: I have carefully reviewed the list of common, wimpy excuses and although I see one or more that I use to justify my current weight situation, I agree that none of them apply to me.

I have entered the "No Excuses Zone"

Action: Make note in your daily journal the top three excuses you have used to justify not starting or staying on a healthy lifestyle program.

Look yourself in the mirror and repeat out loud,
"I have No Excuses!"

Weight Loss for Wimps™
Success Step Eight

<u>Attitude</u>: I acknowledge that emotional eating is a powerful force in my life that must be defeated.

I have consistently struggled with how to effectively deal with my emotions but I am determined to do so without using food.

I have <u>not</u> had a healthy, wholesome relationship with food but am committed to forever changing that relationship.

<u>Skills</u>: I will implement each of the six steps in the *I Learn™ to End Emotional Eating* process.

I will incorporate into my daily life the *I Love™ Good Food Philosophy* to permanently change my relationship with food.

Action: Carefully study the details of the *I Learn*™ process; document the six steps in your daily journal. Begin recording the emotional triggers you encounter over the next few weeks. Make special notes about your successes in implementing these new skills.

Review the *I Love*™ *Good Food* Philosophy on a daily basis. Record these beliefs and attitudes in your journal. Consider posting them on your refrigerator door.

Weight Loss for Wimps™
Success Step Nine

Attitude: I acknowledge that I sometimes don't handle unexpected stressful situations very well and use food to help calm my nerves.

I also acknowledge that I have over-committed some of my time to unnecessary activities that I can live without.

I feel at times that I am overwhelmed.

Skills: When I face an unexpected crisis, I will seek out loving and supporting people who can help me. I will not try to do it alone.

I am committed to simplifying my lifestyle in order to focus on the important tasks. I will eliminate superfluous activities to create blocks of time to relax, relieve stress and to develop healthy eating and exercise habits.

I will say "<u>No</u>" often, with a smile on my face and without guilt.

Action: Make a list in your journal of specific activities that you will eliminate immediately. Be ruthless! Also list those tasks that you can delegate to others or that you can phase out quickly.

Starting today, record in your journal when you said "<u>No</u>".

Make new friends with funny, happy people!

**Weight Loss for Wimps™
Success Step Ten**

Attitude: I acknowledge that I have been unnecessarily fearful of experiencing real hunger.

I now understand that hunger pangs are normal and that I will likely experience them on a daily basis during my weight loss phase and during my future maintenance program.

Skills: I know how to distinguish between real hunger and fake (phantom) hunger.

I will adopt the self-talk *Hunger Is Good™ Mindset* when dealing with real hunger.

I will incorporate high fiber and high-protein foods into my diet, where appropriate, to help combat hunger. I will also use high volume, low calorie soups and salads in my meal planning.
I will implement the *I Learn™* and *I Love Good Food™* techniques for dealing with fake hunger along with…diversion, distraction, movement, activity.

Action: Recalibrate your body and mind to experiencing real hunger for a day. Do not eat anything after breakfast, until the evening meal. Make notes in your personal journal each hour during the day to record your hunger levels (strong, weak, none) and how long any hunger pangs lasted. Drink plenty of water or tea during this test.

Review your notes after dinner to detect any patterns… how many incidents of hunger? How long did they last? Did you survive? Big deal or not a big deal?

**Weight Loss for Wimps™
Success Step Eleven**

Attitude: I now understand that the Western diet is no longer acceptable in my life.

I acknowledge that eliminating junk food from my house and diet must become a top priority that I will implement immediately.

When I see my (formerly) favorite junk food, I will say to myself, *"I don't eat that crap anymore!"*

Skills: I will adopt an eating style that will incorporate clean, fresh vegetables, fruits, lean proteins and whole grains.

I will study, memorize and implement the *10 Abraham Lincoln Eating Rules™*, into my life immediately.

I will estimate my daily calorie intake needs and make necessary adjustments based on actual results. I will record my food consumption in my personal daily log. A free *Weight Loss for Wimps™ Daily Journal* (including a daily food log) is available at:
http://www.wimpdailyjournal.com

Action: Choose an eating style that is compatible with your personal beliefs, philosophy and family values.

Begin researching and collecting recipes for foods that you really like. Make a shopping list for the next week and go shopping.

Decide which day (today?) will be your *Transformation Day* – the first day of your new life and new lifestyle…mark it on your calendar and record it in your personal journal.

Implement and Celebrate!

**Weight Loss for Wimps™
Success Step Twelve**

<u>**Attitude**</u>: Evaluate the attitudes that I have adopted to supplement my eating style and see if any are appropriate for you.

<u>**Skills**</u>: I will develop a set of portion control rules to insure that I will never over eat and will strive to always create a caloric deficit

<u>**Action**</u>: Record in your journal any supplemental attitudes that you will incorporate in your eating rules. I will document my portion control rules and will diligently follow them at every meal.

**Weight Loss for Wimps™
Success Step Thirteen**

<u>**Attitude**</u>: I acknowledge that I have not made physical activity a priority in my daily life; this behavior is no longer acceptable.

My goal is to permanently leave the couch potato lifestyle behind. I have no legitimate excuse for not exercising my body on a daily basis.

Skills: I will adjust my priorities and schedule to incorporate at least 15 minutes of intensive exercise. At a minimum, I will begin walking or swimming.

I will also consider a weight lifting program because I know that it will accelerate my weight loss program and improve my fitness

Action: Decide whether or not you are going to join a local fitness club or are going to work out at home.

Record in your daily journal the type of intensive exercise you did and how you felt afterwards. Do this every day.

Weight Loss for Wimps™
Success Step Fourteen

Attitude: I now understand the importance of holding myself accountable in public. It is extremely powerful, if done correctly.

I also acknowledge that I need to monitor my weight loss progress on a frequent schedule. This will allow me to make instant adjustment to my eating and physical activity levels, as necessary.

Skills: I will carefully consider with whom to share my weight loss program goals and will surround myself with very supportive people.

Action: Decide how often you will weigh yourself (at least weekly) and record your progress in your daily journal.

Decide whether or not you want to bring a fitness trainer and/or a weight loss coach into your life. At least talk to a couple of each before making a final decision.

To contact Kevin Myers or to be placed on a mailing list to receive updates about new releases, visit his website:

http://www.weightloss4wimps.com

ABOUT THE AUTHOR

Kevin Myers is the best-selling author of the real estate investment book, **Buy It, Fix It, Sell It: Profit!** published by Dearborn (Chicago), 2nd edition 2003. This book was the #1 best seller in its category on Amazon and Barnes & Noble. Selected by the Wall Street Journal Online as among the Top 10 real estate investment books of all time.

After college, Kevin and his wife Sharon joined the Peace Corps and served in Cameroon, Africa on a fisheries project. Former Coast Guard officer in Alaska. Environmental manager on projects in Alaska and the Amazon rainforest in Ecuador. Lived in Costa Rica for 4 years.

Kevin lives with his wife Sharon and rescue boxer "Louie" in the North Dallas, Texas area. They have two grown, well educated, beautiful daughters Nicole and Tiffany. Kevin enjoys fly-fishing, golf, riding his Harley and college football (go Sooners!).